Girl on Fire

An Uncommon Love Story

Ana Ramana

Copyright 2016 Ana Ramana

All rights reserved.

ISBN 978-0-9978358-0-9 Paperback

Published by Wild Rose Press

Drawings, pages 6, 136, and 178: Bruce Waldman

Author photo, page 267: Dayna Willbanks

By the same author:

Hymns to the Beloved
The Boy Who Would be Sage
Taf

Dedication

*For every girl or boy, woman or man
who has suffered at the hands
of sexual or physical abuse*

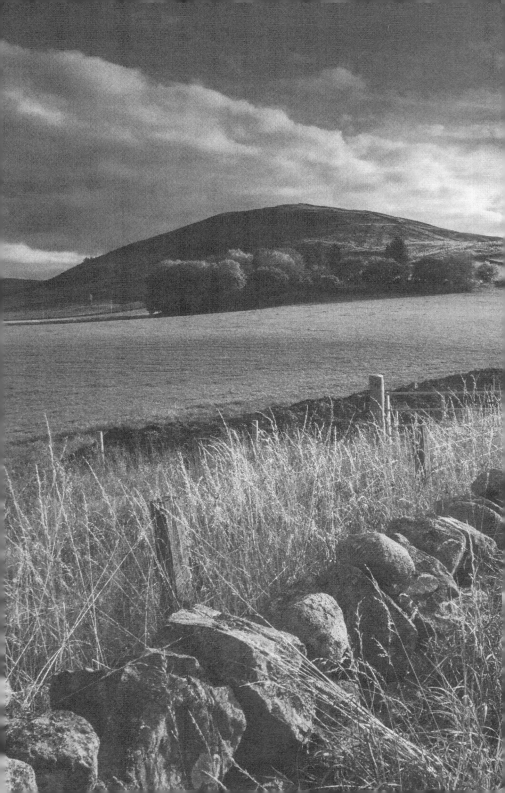

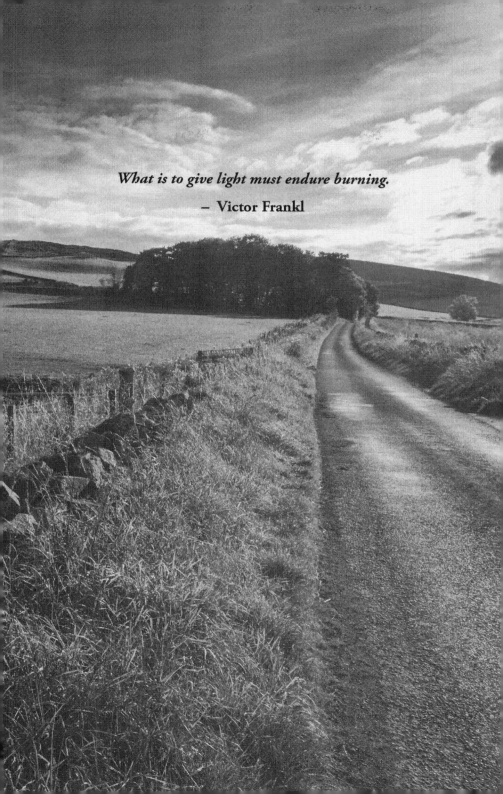

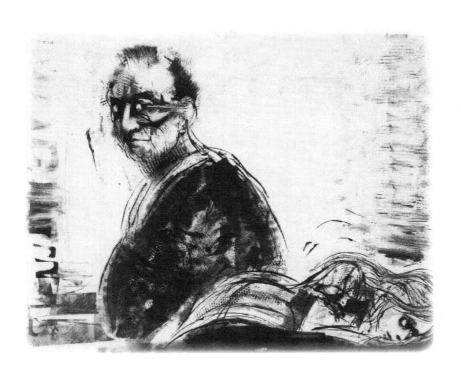

Book 1

IRELAND

I see myself
on the underworld side of that water,
the darkness coming in fast, saying
all the names I know for a lost land:
Ireland. Absence. Daughter.

– Eavan Boland

Prologue

When she first plunged into that dark womb, she could still hear them singing through the stars to her. She was a sphere of throbbing light, radiating. Silver sparks flew off her and filled the cave of her new home. The imprint of her life was already graven, she could see it unfurl before her, helpless now to change anything. But still she trusted, even as the black wetness smeared her being, even as the heaving rains of Ireland crowded round that vessel carrying her. She tasted her first bite of loneliness. This mother walking through the world with her in tow; all she could do was follow. And still they sang, messengers from her true home, filling the void with beauty, with a soft light if she could just keep her attention on it.

Voices rose and fell beyond the walls of her room, heavy, hard syllables she could barely understand. It seemed a strange language, devoid of the brimming heart of love she knew she was. How had she ended up here? Had she chosen this?

Sometimes she felt a light tapping outside the mother's body.

"She's there, Missus!"

"I heard her move!"

Yes, she was restless, rocking her tiny limbs in the gray fluid, to ease the new feelings passing through her. From where did they come? Whose were they? Foreign they felt, and she an alien sprouting arms and legs in this new country. Who was the mother to her? Or she to the mother?

Sometimes it felt hard to breathe – a kind of smoke billowing around the tissues of her home. She sipped drizzles of air and followed the mother's movements, the singing floating from further off, she who had never known distance or time.

Let love be my home, she thought, let all that unfolds melt into that. She consoled herself, made it her mission to always hold close the truth that was her familiar. To let this life wash through her like a pure river, and breathe, simply breathe.

Never forget who you are, they sang to her from afar.

And as she inched painfully through that barrier of flesh into another kind of darkness, she made her covenant.

EAMON

Helpless, he was, to resist. All this love, or was it passion, gushing up inside him, an eternity of tears, and who else could receive it if not her? She could save him. *Lord, be my salvation.* Well, much good that prayer had done him. Let her be his savior. She wanted to, just look at that face, wide open like the sun in summer, beaming just for him. She wanted it too, surely she did. She could take his heartache, she was so, well, empty, like there was nothing inside her, only light. There was room there, surely, ample room, for his hurting heart.

He didn't even feel the zip of his trousers opening, or the swollen bruise slide out with his hands. His head was far off in a dream land where nothing bad ever happened. In a flash, though there was no time really, this was outside of time, her mouth was wedged open like a chalice waiting for him, her baby teeth barely formed, grazing the skin of his flesh. It felt electric, a hundred bees thrumming, a light searing through his head, her coughing, and the slow leak of a gummy milk down her chin, her bib full of it, of him, of his love for her, he hoped she knew that. It was only love, pure and simple, their secret church, a marriage made in heaven.

He tucked himself back in, wiped the scum off her face with the sleeve of his shirt, his body a sea of rough waves still, cold, even in the August heat. Her spluttering would ease up soon, and she'd sleep then, dreaming of his warmth on her silvery tongue.

Amen, he sighed, as he made the Sign of the Cross, and went on his collection rounds for the parish Planned Giving.

EILY

The roads were icy as her mother dragged her along by the hand after Mass.

"Hurry now, Eily," her mother shouted through the searing wind. "The turkey has to be in the oven for three hours. What kind of Christmas would it be without a turkey?"

Liquid dripped from Eily's nose as she scuttled along, wondering if it would freeze on her face. Her gloves were threadbare. Eily's mother plucked a white hanky from her handbag. It had violets embroidered on the edges. Grandma in England always sent one for Christmas. "Let me wipe you up, child. You look like the wreck of the Hesperus!"

The bleached cotton tugged at her face while Eily shivered.

"Ah, Mrs. Annesley! Happy Christmas to you!"

Eily squinted her face up to find Mrs. Annesley walking towards them. Her head was drooping as if it was too heavy to hold up. She had a young boy by the hand. Eily felt she didn't want to talk to her mother.

"Sure, it's not such a great Christmas, Missus."

"And why in heavens not?"

Eily's heart lurched in her chest as she watched Mrs. Annesley collapse into tears.

"What's the matter?" Her mother's voice softened and reached out an arm towards the weeping woman.

"Santy didn't come." Her shoulders heaving up and down.

"Oh…" Eily rarely saw her mother speechless but she had her arm on the weeping woman's shoulder. "Oh… I'm so sorry."

Eily started to feel angry at Santy. Why would he visit some houses and skip theirs? Didn't he know there was a child inside? She couldn't believe the boy, skinny and forlorn looking, had been so bad that he'd be ignored by Santy, who was supposed to be almost a saint.

She glanced into the boy's pale green eyes before he looked down in a way that you'd swear the cracked footpath held the answers to every problem.

As her mother dragged her down the avenue, clucking at the strangeness of this world, Eily decided she'd give the boy her present, whatever it was.

When she unwrapped the heavy box under the tree, carefully undoing the pink ribbon, she found a little washing machine. It had a plastic door you pulled out, where you were supposed to put in the clothes, and she fiddled with the dials until it started to make a noise like a car warming up. Then it shook as if it were out in the cold without a coat. Eily decided there and then never to become a housewife like her mother, where you were endlessly filling and emptying a machine.

Was Santy trying to tell her she was dirty? No, she decided. She thought maybe the boy with green eyes could use it to prop his soldiers on, though who knew if he even had any.

She tip toed into Liam's room and plucked a few plastic soldiers out of the cardboard box in the corner. Carefully she wrapped each of them in the Christmas paper and put them inside the machine as a surprise and she let herself out the back door, shivering, as she raced down to Annesley's and put the machine on the front step beside the empty milk bottles.

"Santy," she scolded the air, "next year, you better bring something better for that sad boy, or for me, so I can give it to him. Or I'll never, ever write to you again."

She was growing up now, almost forty inches tall. They measured every girl in Eily's class, the back wall a zigzag of black marks where everyone had stood under a ruler and Sister Carmelita had stitched a pencil across their height. She may have been almost six but she still loved to teach the flowers in O'Reilly's garden next door. She knew, really, that they had no need to learn anything but she couldn't help reeling off all the rivers of Ireland, *Liffey, Lee, Bann, Suir,* once she'd memorized them, and then the mountain ranges, and the four provinces. Any little bit of special knowledge she tucked into her brain, she would save until she got to the row of daffodils lined up like eager pupils on O'Reilly's lawn, and in she would skip, up close to them, and with her ruler or pencil, she'd run through the list like a headmaster, *Leinster, Ulster, Munster, Connaught,* pointing at a different flower for each province.

She had to be careful because Mrs. O'Reilly came home from her job at Glady's Hair Salon on the half past five. Mr. was always at some park or other, where he was superintendent, until very late at night. Eily had the garden to herself after school. And the flowers loved her. The light seeping through every petal lit up her heart. They had no dark edges or insides, like people, and they wanted nothing more than to please you, to share their beauty with you, without reward.

Eily would congratulate them on their gaining height or the curve of a particular stem, sometimes she would stoop over and kiss them, or run her tongue along the groove of a petal. She savored the sun shining through them, so gauzy you could almost cup the gleaming light in your own hands.

When February went to sleep and March woke slowly up, Eily's mother hired Jim to help in the garden. He came from the rough part of town, wore a gray jacket with holes in the elbows. He barely spoke two words, and only to mumble, but Eily saw the bright light streaming out of his heart and she loved him.

He seemed a giant to her, so tall he was, and thin as a broom handle but she would follow him around, helping to pull up weeds and clear away wind-strewn branches. Sometimes he'd hoosh her up high and swing her in circles, her braids winging through the air like little birds. She loved the smell of him, all dirt and twigs and leaves. A few times, he'd rustle a clove drop out of his jacket pocket like a magician. He'd let her kneel down with him in the grass and hand her weeds for their pile. He was careful with his long, lumbering hands, treating each stalk of dead grass as if it was royalty.

When her mother had to go to England to look after her own mother and her father off at work, Jim walked Eily the quarter mile to school and waved her off with hand blown kisses. He pulled out a soiled hanky from his trousers pocket and raised it in the air, a gift specially for her. She could still see the dark white cotton blowing in the breeze as she entered the convent gates.

She struggled with her uniform, the navy blue costume that held all her parts in. She felt strapped into it and the nuns were forever chiding her for her dickey bow being askew or her socks falling down, what with the elastic gone out of them. She was supposed to have a pair of indoor and outdoor shoes but there wasn't the money so she wore the same Clark's runners everywhere. The girls in her class would tie her shoelaces together to make her trip but Eily didn't care. She just thought about Jim and counted the minutes until school was over.

She'd take Jim to O'Reilly's and sit him down in the flower bed next to the tulips and she'd teach them all she'd learned in school that day. She'd do a dance for her quiet audience and the wind would wave in applause.

After the last lesson, Eily raced out the school gate, her school bag banging against her leg. He was leaning against the wall and she took off at a belt to meet the arms opening towards her, only to be intercepted by Sister Carmelita.

"Where do you think you're going, child?"

"Home. With Jim."

Eily watched as Sister Carmelita surveyed the scrawny man standing at the gate. She took Eily by the wrist and said, "You'll not be going anywhere with him."

"But it's Jim, my friend! He's come to take me home."

"We shall see about that, young Miss. And you, sir, if you're looking for handouts, we only give food to the poor on Thursdays."

Jim took off his cap, opened his mouth and closed it again. Eily watched him turn round and slink back up the avenue, his head hung low.

"Jim! Jim!"

He turned back with a sad smile and said, "It's no use, Eily."

Eily tried to wrench her wrist out of the nun's firm grip to no avail.

"We can't have you being accosted by tramps while your mother's away," was all she said before marching Eily back to her classroom to sit and wait and weep.

EAMON

He couldn't help himself, the radio blaring the big news of the day. It must be a sign, he told himself. And before he could bless himself, he'd made an illegal U-turn, shunned the office and headed north again. Let someone else trawl the houses and try to pawn off insurance on unwitting souls. Sure, he'd not be missed, would he? And even if he was, he'd say he'd gotten another migraine. The girl'd be out of school in ten minutes, he'd better get a move on. The green lights egged him on and he got to the convent gates with a minute to spare.

He watched the girls in their navy uniforms swinging their satchels as they sauntered out in groups to the road. Where was she? He checked his watch. They'd barely make it in time. Five minutes. Ten. He loosened his tie. Ah, there she was, straggling down the long driveway, bending down every few seconds to touch a flower. What was she doing at all, the cratúr? Much as he loved her, the light blue of her eyes, her soft smile, he had to admit she'd a few strange ways about her.

When she saw him, she looked surprised, faltered a moment before waving.

"Da! What're you doing here? Shouldn't you be at work?"

"I've the day off, Eily. Hop in!"

The girl slid into the seat beside him, clutching her school bag in her lap.

"I've a surprise for you, child. We're going somewhere very special."

His heart tweaked a bit, seeing the joy in her face. She was so easy to please, unlike the wife. Or even Liam. No one seemed satisfied with their lives, always moaning about this or that. But the girl never complained, only offered the warmth of her heart to whoever she came across.

"Oh Da! Where to?"

He wasn't sure how to broach it. She was still young but wouldn't it do them both a power of good to get a blessing from on high. Sure, they'd not have the chance again.

"We're going to see the car..." but the word caught in his throat. He coughed, "...ival."

"The carnival? Really?" Eily twitched in her seat with delight. "You mean with a Big Top and candy floss and dodgems...?"

"You'll see, girl. Just be quiet now and we'll get there faster." He noticed Eily squirming in her seat, as if she didn't quite believe him. If he drove a bit faster, maybe she'd settle down. Sure, it would be a bit of a carnival all right, a feast day to recall for years to come. He took off his tie.

"Ah, Santry. We're almost here."

A crowd was gathering on the avenue in front of a tall stage. As they got out of the car, Eily asked, "Where are all the children?"

"They'll be along, girl, you'll see," He'd almost convinced himself she'd enjoy this as much as any carnival. What better privilege than this could there be?

He took the girl's hand and led her through the throngs to the front of the stage. A man with tufts for hair was talking into a microphone. "And it is with great pleasure that I hand you over now to none other than his Eminence, Cardinal Conway."

Eily watched as a round man, dressed head to toe in red, wearing a wizard's steepled hat, shuffled out onto the stage.

She looked up at her father, eyes brimming. "It's not a carnival at all, is it?"

"Now, now," he was occupied, releasing her hand from his and making the sign of the cross.

Eily looked at all the old people blessing themselves and half bowing, not a child in sight, and she turned on her heels and marched back, eyes stinging, towards the car.

EILY

Eily felt all grown up when her mother sent her up to Whitty's to buy a box of Persil. She wondered if it would have worked in the washing machine she'd given the boy down the road. But he wouldn't have needed it, anyway. "Oh dear," her mother had picked in her purse. "Not enough for mixed veg, I'm afraid. Just the detergent, Eileen, please."

Mr. Whitty helped Eily count out the change down to the last sixpence. "Tell your mother I was asking for her," he shouted after Eily. "A real lady, she is."

As she was coming down the avenue, Eily couldn't help pausing by Colonel Timmons' house. He had the biggest garden in the parish, long rows of vegetables bursting out of the earth and a cluster of bright flowers in one corner. Eily inhaled the beauty a moment and before she knew it, she'd legged it over the wall and tugged a huge cabbage out of the ground. It was purple as the evening sky. She clutched it like a prized football all the way home, trying to decide how she'd explain the gift to her mother.

"Here, Ma," Eily set the goods on the kitchen table.

"Mum! When will you ever learn to call me by my proper name?" her mother chided. "Go out and play now so I can… Where did this come from?"

Eily held up the round prize, her face beaming. "Mr. Whitty sent it for you. He was asking after you."

Her mother slid a curl away from her face, smiling. "Well, well, isn't that grand." She lifted it up and spun it around. "It's fresh as if it was only just plucked! I must run up there tomorrow and thank him personally."

"Sure, there's no need." Eily hadn't imagined she might be caught out in her lie. "He said it was to be a secret."

"Secret? Why on earth?"

Eily scarpered out the back door, the wind whistling behind her.

Next day, when Eily came home from school, her father was waiting in the kitchen. His voice loud and sharp, he said stealing was a sin, that you'd never get to heaven if you took things that didn't belong to you. It didn't matter even if you intended good, it was a black mark against you and it might take years in Purgatory for being so brazen and bold.

"Go to your room now, girl," he nudged her up the stairs. "And don't come down till we're ready for the Rosary."

Ugly was Liam's name for her. She didn't mind because sometimes her brother'd tickle her under the arms and she'd roll around on the torn carpet laughing. Mostly though, he had a look of gloom on his face, especially after reading about the war of Independence. He was obsessed with it.

He held court at supper talking about Nelson's Pillar and how the Irish were mad for having a statue of an English admiral on the main street of the country they'd oppressed. "It won't last long there, let me tell you," he said.

"May I remind you that your own mother is English, Liam?"

"Yeah well, maybe there's the odd good one."

"And not a few good looking ones either," Eily's mother laughed and pointed at her chiffon blouse.

"Better than anyone else I've seen in an apron!" Liam always knew the right thing to say.

He'd been to O'Connell Street, just out of curiosity, and he said that once you climbed to the top, you had a view for miles. Eily pictured blue sky, a platform she could step out on and be within kissing distance of the angels.

She begged him to take her. "Just this once, would you?"

"Sure, how would I get you back home? I've lectures on the south side."

"Pleeease. I'll walk home."

"You'd never find your way. It costs, you know, you can't just get in free."

They bartered back and forth, Eily's mother even taking her side, until Liam caved in.

"All right. But wrap up warm and make sure you have bus fare home."

So Eily rode into town on the crossbar of her brother's bicycle. The March wind tore at her hair but she leaned into it, a smile splitting her face in half. They zoomed down the Washerwoman's Hill, even passed the 19 bus, and on beyond The Botanics, Phibsboro, The Bohemian cinema, and onto Parnell Street. The tips of Eily's fingers were puce but her heart was light. She was going on an adventure.

She slid off the bar once they got to O'Connell Street. Liam's cheeks were almost raw. She marveled that her brother would have eyes shaped like upturned wings, so different from hers. He came from underneath a different cabbage leaf, her mother had explained. It must have been from China or somewhere, Eily mused, as she watched her brother wind a padlock around his bike. She wanted eyes like his so much she'd tried to pull them back with her hair clips but got an infection instead.

Oliver Twist was playing at the Corinthian across the road. They walked past the Gresham Hotel, oh, it looked fancy. How she'd love a warm mug of cocoa there on those plush seats.

On they went until they came to the Pillar. Eily hadn't imagined it to be so tall. It seemed to jut up into the sky, slicing it in two.

Liam pointed up. "You've a bird's eye view all the way to the sea from the top."

"Oh! I've been wishing for ages to see the ocean!"

There was a short queue of people ahead of them but the closer they got, the more Eily's breath quickened. It seemed to leap about in her chest. She stood behind her brother as he placed his change on the kiosk counter.

Inside it was dark except for a strand of bulbs wandering up the round stairway. The walls were the color of dust, patches black as their coal house. It felt cold and smelled of sweaty socks. Eily's throat glutted.

"I'll race you to the top." Liam legged it up the steps, eager to go. Eily stood stock still, glued to the ground beneath her. She heard Liam grunting as he came back down towards her.

"Don't be a babby now," he took her hand, dragging her behind him, Eily holding back, a taut line between them.

They took a few steps before Eily crouched against the wall.

"C'monnn, Ugly, it's only another hundred steps or so."

But Eily wouldn't budge. They watched as a young boy and his father passed them. "What's wrong with yer one?" The man asked.

"Listen, I paid three pence to get you in. We're not stopping now…"

"I can't."

"You were the one begged me to come. *Pleeeease, Liam, pleeeeese.*"

He was making fun of her. She lurched onto another step but her stomach was all bound up and she thought she might vomit.

She leaned into the black wall, Liam leering at her.

"What're you so afraid of?"

When she closed her eyes, she could see the little cupboard under the stairs at home where they kept the vacuum and shoe polish. She'd said something she shouldn't, hadn't she, and someone had shoved her into that dark cave. She'd been trapped, alone, screaming in the dark to no one. When she opened her eyes, it was black as night, and she didn't know which was worse, there or here.

"I'm… not… able."

Liam tried yanking on her arm again but she couldn't move, only pulled against him, shaking.

Her brother heaved a long sigh and turned them around towards the entrance.

"Youse weren't long in there," the man at the kiosk said. Liam ignored him.

"Don't you ever ask me to take you anywhere again, d'ye hear me?"

Eily nodded.

"And you owe me three P."

She took big gulps of fresh air, glad to be out in the open, cupping her eyes against the shock of light, and shivered in the wind all the way to the bus stop.

All week, Eily tried to make sense of that black fear that had shrouded her. What had she said that was so terrible? Why couldn't she remember? Only the tight knot in her throat and the door slamming behind her. That night, after her father said his usual good night, she lay in bed imagining herself taking the Pillar steps in two's, alongside her brother, not a hint of hesitation in her. One day, she'd have the courage to go again, she would surely.

Only a day or two passed when Liam lashed in the back door at tea time. He had the Irish Press under his arm. "Turn on the news! You won't believe it."

Eily and her mother looked at him.

"They're after blowing it up!" His voice was high and his breath jagged.

"What?"

"The Pillar! I knew it! The IRA gave Nelson the old what for!"

Eily's mother turned on the radio. "In a surprise attack early this morning, the tallest statue in Dublin was blown to smithereens. One man was injured. There are conflicting reports as to who was responsible but many are pointing to the Irish Republican Army. Until further notice, O'Connell Street is closed to the public."

Eily felt a twinge of sadness that she'd not let herself float up to the crown of the Pillar. Now she would never have a chance again. But Liam was on a tear, she'd not seen him so cheery in a long time. "Good on ye, IRA!" He held the newspaper in the air, like it was a medal of victory or something.

Her mother put the fried eggs on a plate and said, "What on earth is this country coming to?"

Maybe she'd been half asleep, those images of the tower floating like a ghost around her. She'd opened her eyes, all bleary in the violet haze of morning, and there it was at the foot of her bed. The Face hovering again. She'd seen it before. A face of such kindness it made her heart swell, as if she had to grow to make room for it. And it was more than kindness, more even than love, or at least the love she'd known so far. The eyes seemed to carry it, luminous like a billion stars winking at you all at once. There was a heat in it and a lightness that set her skin sparkling. And it seemed to wash all her worries away. And oh, the color of those eyes, they were beyond anything Eily could fathom.

She rubbed her cheeks and shook her head to make sure she was awake. Every time, the vision would last only a few seconds but to Eily, it felt an eternity, like the chalice of her heart was filled to overflowing, brimming with a delight far beyond this world.

What should I do, Face? she whispered into the air. *It's strange to be so afraid of dark places when nothing has really scared me before. I must've said something terrible to be thrown into the cupboard with the vacuum.*

Eily closed her eyes and waited for an answer but it was always the same: after a while, the cold world would descend and she'd crawl out of bed, shivering, but the feeling would stay with her sometimes all day.

She told no one about the Face. Who could she tell? They'd only ignore her or laugh, the way they'd jeered when she spoke of sometimes seeing light in people. Only last week she'd been up at Whitty's with her mother and a boy on crutches hobbled in to get a newspaper for his father, who was leaning against the wall outside, dragging on a Sweet Afton. Eily knew the smell, it reminded her of winter days and all the chimneys whispering of wispy smoke. The boy hadn't enough change for the paper and Mary the assistant was getting cross with him.

"Oh please give it to us," he was almost begging, a smile plastered on his thin face. "Me da'll kill me if I leave without the winner of Spot-The-Ball."

"Tell yer da to try the bookies. There's better odds there," Mary said.

Eily wanted to give him the extra bob but she had nothing and her mother was busy weighing flour. She blew him a kiss from inside her and suddenly an avalanche of pain shook at her heart. She could feel, oh God, she could feel how sad the poor lad was. There was no money to give but she was glad to share in his sadness.

When Eily mentioned it to her mother as they went into Dugan the butcher's, she got a clip on her hand and was told never to mention such foolishness again.

His hands, the heft and softness of them, how he held them out like treasures, dangling above her small body before inching in to the hem of her dress. She'd gone along with her father to Mass even though she didn't have to yet. It was still eleven months to her Communion Day. The flickering light in the red candle holders seemed to whisper to her, *You're safe now, Eily. Just rest.*

And for a while, she had, letting the prayers of the parishioners wash over her, watching the sea of people queueing up to offer their tongues for the Eucharist. That's what it was called, her father said, God's body. At every Mass in the world, he'd cut himself into small, thin rounds so there'd be a taste for everybody.

God must be very generous, Eily thought, and she decided that Father Lamb, a kind of stand-in for God, must be too. So she'd convinced her father to let her visit the priest after Mass. Maybe he could help her piece together the puzzle of her memories.

Father Lamb had looked her up and down at the sacristy door and said, "Good enough, Eamon. I'll take her from here."

"Right-o," her father almost bowed, quietly closing the door as he left.

"I was wondering, Father," she began, "about this thing I might've said that made someone angry so they hid me…"

Father Lamb slid each finger out of his long white gloves like a ballerina, Eily thought.

"Ah now," his words dripped out slowly, "you should never say anything to upset another, should you?"

Eily wasn't certain. Wasn't it more important not to tell lies? When she didn't respond, the priest said, "As my own mother, Lord have mercy on her, used say, 'If you can't say anything good, don't say anything at all.'"

And then his hands, almost in slow motion, opening before her like a fan. Fingers snaked up her scrawny, mottled legs, a dozen spiders half-tickling, half-torturing her. And when he unearthed that fresh meadow, spreading the skin like a knife slicing an envelope, she caught her breath, held it in as long as she could, but still the water came teeming out, streaming over his fine, unworked palms, an odyssey of blinding light.

"Mother of God," he yelled. "What the jaysus are you doing, girl?"

She hunched the froth of her skirt in close to her, her entire being aquiver.

Nothing. That's what she said. Nothing, just like her father waiting outside, on his knees, head tilted towards the heavens, hands clasped at his chest like lost wings.

The door opened abruptly. "Here she is, take her, Eamon. And away with you both."

"Oh thank you, Father, thank you. C'mon now, Eily. It's almost tea time."

She let him take her pale hand in his, all ruddy and rough, bristling against her thumb. Her legs were still wet, dribbles leaking down to her knees. She could feel a drop slowly floating inside her sock, a ray of sun streaking round her ankles. How could her father not notice, she wondered, as they huddled under a torn umbrella, fighting rain on the long walk home.

"He wants to see you again." Eily's father wiped the rain off his mac when he came in after the 8 o'clock.

"Why?"

"Lord knows. You should be grateful a man of his stature'd be offering spiritual counsel to you so young."

She tried coughing, saying she wasn't well but her father would have none of it. Maybe he only wanted to say sorry or maybe she should, she didn't know. But she decided she wouldn't let fear get the best of her this time. She'd be prepared. Before she left, she folded five strips of toilet paper into her gabardine pocket and told her father she wanted to use the loo before he took her back to the sacristy. He let her, but said, "Hurry up now, Eily. You've a man of the cloth waiting on you."

He had a cloth squeezed tight between his hands when she arrived. Her heart thundered in her chest yet she couldn't help but walk towards him.

"Bend over," he told her, without as much as a greeting. "And I'll give you what's good for you."

She made a C of her tiny body as he tore at her girl pants, and as the whipping and the fingers came at her in such a flurry, she couldn't make out what was pleasure or pain. Only a wild fire in her lower parts, roaring flames in her throat, an animal on top of her, inside her, rupturing something she hadn't known existed until now, until she became the fire, glowing with the light of God, burning up every known thing, until she felt well and truly singed, until she rose up out of all that ash into vast, open space, and a charm of angels choiring their special tune to her, over and over.

"Girl like you should spend her days in Confession." He shouted after her as she shuffled towards the chapel, into her father's arms and out the back door, a votive candle flickering against the wall like a ghost in their wake.

Eily's mother always had the kettle going. Tea for breakfast, dinner, supper, and every hour in between. Eily didn't like the tarry taste of it, but made herself take it onto her tongue, like she imagined communion, the sheer strength of it washing any sins, any memory, clean away.

    Her father sat in the corner, arms slumped on the kitchen table, slurping out of his huge mug. Eily sometimes thought it was intended for a giant, so tall and broad it was, but he never left a drop remaining.

    "Time for the Rosary," he'd say, soon as the dishes were cleared away. "Pull down the beads, Eily, will you?" And he'd light a candle, shuffle onto his knees, she close by his side, as he began the long, slow, labored incantation, she mimicking his words, head bowed over the stool, the angels whistling on the wind all the while through the cracked window.

    Mother never joined them. She said the English don't believe in prayer and why should they, the world being the way it is. She scrubbed the tea things clean and set them by the sink to drain. The running water sounded like a magic river to Eily's ears as she knelt, trying hard to marry the tap water to that First Sorrowful Mystery, The Agony of Child Jesus in the Garden.

    After the long litanies during which Eily traveled to Medjugorje hoping for a glimpse of Our Lady, which she'd learned about in school, and back, her father would boil the kettle and fill three hot water bottles. Hers was red and smelled of mold, but she loved that it got tucked between the sheets like a special prize waiting for her when she crawled into bed.

    The damp flannel her mother used to wipe her face reminded her of Father Lamb's cloth. It made her whole face pucker, rough edges scouring her cheeks. She slipped into her gossamer nightie as her mother drove a comb through the tangles of her hair.

    In bed, she waited. He'd come up to see her, sure as moonrise. Every night it was the same, he'd make a big fuss of saying goodnight to his wife, yawn like a great big bear, and she knew by the creaks on the stair how close he was. She'd have her light out, lids closed, but in he'd come regardless, and slap down on the counterpane, his breath sometimes cabbage, sometimes rashers. She'd play a game, trying to guess what smell he'd carry on him before he got through the door. When she was right, she'd give herself a gold star in the copy book she kept under the mattress.

Always, he'd start into a ballad, and off he'd go, as if he belonged to the Vienna Boys' Choir, long and sonorous, and all the while, he'd be guiding her girl fingers down the zipper of his trousers, and into that place that grew from attention, and on he'd croon, *The Mountains of Mourne sweep down to the sea…*, scrunching her fingers inside his, close as a kiss, until the fountain came.

"Da," she'd asked him. "Where does all that foam come from?"

"The same place as babies do." Her father tucking himself back in. Eily was fascinated.

"But why do you moan when it drips out like that?"

"Ah sure, sometimes it hurts to have children." Her father sighed. "But not you, you're my special cailín. That's why we have our very own special secret."

"Does Father Lamb make babies…?" Eily began but her father cut her off.

"Enough talk now. It's more like a prayer if we work in silence." And he lurched out of the room, almost breathless. "Sleep tight."

So many secrets, Eily sighed. If she ever had babies, she'd keep nothing from them.

When she was wrong, she'd pry out a strand of her hair and put it under her pillow.

After he'd gone, she'd wait until the house was calm, before slipping out from under the covers and tiptoeing downstairs, skipping over the creaks, her feet bathed in light, until she reached the back door. Unlatching it, she stepped out into the cold, dark air, her feet stiffening on the frosty patch of grass in the garden. And she'd pull off her nightie, swipe the smear off her palms, and lift her face skywards. She loved to imagine the moon smiling down on her bare, shivering flesh as she twirled her arms and swung her hipbones this way and that, making mad circles, head spinning, hair loosed and flying, until she filled to the brim with wild light, until there was no she, no father, no mother, no priest, only stars flowing through that vast space, until she became the cosmos itself.

She came from the angels, she knew it in her bones and sinew. She knew she had wings that could take her anywhere, away from this foreign soil where people kept their lips sealed against truth, where they looked down or away, not all the way through to the flower of your heart. She knew that no matter the bleak landscape, the harsh bodies, the brutal, wandering fingers, that she was safe. Nothing could touch her, though she had been touched and more. Nothing could stain who she really was. She knew her friend, The Face, shawled her every move, that her mother and father were borrowed, sad, lost creatures who somehow needed her in ways she could not understand. She knew she could never speak of this; it was her special secret, the one she cleaved close to her chest, the one that made her every single breath worthwhile.

In the blueblack of morning, she came down to the smell of polish and all the shoes lined up like school children in the washroom, gleaming like a brand new day. And he bent over the hearth, blowing smoke into the newspapers and piled twigs, ashes dancing in stars all around him.

It was her favorite time, watching her father do what she imagined adults in every house up and down the road do. Getting everything in place, plates, spoons, sugar on the table, milk in the pitcher, curtains drawn back. The whole world a normal place where she could spoon porridge out of the pot like every other girl she knew, waiting for her mother, and almost belong.

"Mum," Eily tugged at her mother's apron. "Can I tell you something?"

Her mother was kneading dough on the kitchen table. "What is it, Eileen? Can't you see I'm busy? It's almost lunch time and the bread's not even in the oven yet."

"Father Lamb…?"

"What about him?"

"Do all priests use their fingers to explore parts of…?"

"Damnation!" The bowl of flour tipped over and a cascade of soft dust drizzled to the floor. "Not now, child. I haven't the time."

Eily bent over to help clean up the mess and cracked heads with her mother. "Just leave!" her mother barked. "I can do it myself!"

Slinking out of the kitchen, Eily went upstairs and pulled out her copy book from under the bed. She scrawled her pencil across the first page, tears splashing the paper. If no one would listen, she'd just dream up her own world where people would sit you on their lap and say, softly, *Eily love, why don't you share your troubles to your heart's content?*

Liam stumbled into the kitchen one afternoon with a dog in his arms. "Found him in the bushes by the quarry. He's nobody's."

Eily took one look at the little creature, his tail going like a see saw, and fell fast in love. He looked around the kitchen quickly before hiding under the table and scarpered out the back door as soon as he could.

"Bollox!" Liam said. "He's ran away from me twice. Had to carry him home by his scruff."

"Watch your language!" Eily's mother said.

Liam called him Banjo because he said the creature was a gypsy, couldn't settle in any one place. When he did stay home, Eily would spend hours out the back, Banjo by her side, stroking and singing him songs she'd learned in school. When he licked her face until it was a river of saliva, she'd lick him back, delighted. He was the best thing that had happened to her in all of her seven years. Sometimes they'd make sausage rolls of their bodies and spin around on the damp grass. Soon Banjo followed her everywhere.

Eily would wave him goodbye from the front gate as she left for school and she'd count the hours until she could get home again to see her new friend. If he'd been left outside, Banjo would be waiting on the road and race to meet her, his tail at full throttle.

Sometimes he'd sit by the swing on his haunches while she soared in the air, singing to both of them and no one in particular. Banjo was a song in her heart.

EAMON

That Willy, he'd give him what for one of these days, who cares if he was the senior salesman. Thinking he has all the answers to the ills of this world, as if murdering babies was the cure-all. Lord alone knows, he was liberal himself in ways. Sure, didn't the Communists have it right, sharing the wealth with no one left out. They had a pride in being poor, just like Jesus himself. So why did Willy have to make his life hell just because he passed the picket? For God's sake, he wasn't going to put his good name behind the innocent slaughter of children.

But Willy's taunts wouldn't leave him as he drove home, the girl in the back seat. It brought to mind the boys' jeers when he was a lad, trying to save the birds they'd be tossing rocks at. Feckin' messers. Sure, what was the use? If Willy had his way, and he was related to the general manager, he'd be out of a job in no time. Bad cess to him anyway.

The car scraped against the rusted gate pulling into the drive. He hadn't been thinking, hadn't judged the angle right. "Bloody gate!" He yelled and braked the car. "Out with you, Eily. Out now!"

And he'd hardly a foot outside the car door before Banjo was nipping at his heel. "G'way from me, y'eejit. I'm warning you."

"Daddy! It's only Banjo saying welcome home."

"Get off me, you little gurrier!" But the dog kept jumping up on his leg, his only suit covered in dirt. He hefted his boot high above the dog. "Don't say I didn't warn you!" and rammed the butt of his heel into the dog's back. You couldn't believe the squealing.

"Daddy! Daddy!" Now Eily was crying, chasing after the critter under the bushes. "How could you?"

He didn't know which was worse, to stay there and watch his girl sobbing or head into the house and her with only mean comments for him. He shook his head, surprised at the might of his mood, and skulked indoors.

EILY

Eily wandered the roads, looking through a window here or there, wondering if the angels ever visited any of those lonely people inside. She was beginning to understand how sad this planet was, how leached of light. Where had it all gone when once it had shone through every single thing? She came to the edge of the estate, where what her mother called the ruffians lived. She knew big fights happened here, gangs with knives and iron bars and they wouldn't have a second thought about knocking you sideways with one.

Banjo had disappeared again. It always made her heart miss a beat when he was gone, praying it wouldn't be the last time she saw the love of her life. She'd looked everywhere she could think of and no sight of him. Maybe she'd run into Jim up here. He'd help her find him, she knew he would.

It was almost night when she stopped, just stood on the path, no idea where to go next. So she stood and listened to the sound of her breathing, light and shallow, hardly there. She thought she might never move again.

And then she heard it, a voice rising out of the air, a man's voice. She found him sitting on a patch of grass in front of the quarry.

"Just wait a few years," he said, taking a long, slow draw on a cigarette.

She recognized him, good looking, maybe twenty or so, collar of his leather jacket hunched round his neck. She'd seen many a girl on his arm.

On Raglan road, on an autumn day, I saw her first and knew, he was almost singing, *that her red hair would weave a snare that I might one day rue...*

Eily stared at him as if he were from another planet. He made no move to touch her.

"Don't ye know Kavanagh's poem?" he half-whispered,

squishing his cigarette butt with his polished shoe. "One day you'll make mince meat of mens' hearts, young one, and it'll make sense to ye then."

Eily eyed him in the dim light. His face seemed to shapeshift. One second, he'd look like her father, the next, Father Lamb. Eily blinked hard, trying to bring back the man she'd first seen. But now everything melted into that warm, gentle Face that seemed to be composed only of light. He could have jumped on her but all he'd done was be kind. Eily wondered if she'd imagined it but then she heard a deep cough; it was him walking away.

Eily wobbled slowly back the way she had come, something coming to life again within her. The poem could have been in double dutch but each word falling out of his mouth was like a magic charm. She could have listened to him half singing forever. One day she would make music of words herself.

An almost stranger he'd been but surely it was a message from the heavens that things would turn out right in the end.

When she'd almost finished the long walk home, she felt a wet tongue on her leg. "Banjo! You scared the life out of me. I was in bits thinking you'd left me." She hunkered down and ruffled his fur. She felt the elastic in her pants snap as she moved. Good riddance, she smiled, as she let them pool round her ankles and stepped out of them, "Then what would I do, tell me? Let's go, Banjo. You're all I'll ever need."

Next day, when she was chasing Banjo round the garden, Eily was stopped in her tracks by a fierce tightening in her stomach. She clutched at it, trying to staunch the pain but she couldn't and fell onto the grass, roiling around like a poisoned animal, screaming to high heaven with all her might.

It was Mrs. Gallagher who found her, heard her from the street, and she took one look at Eily and said, "Holy Mother! I'm ringing for an ambulance now, so I am."

The hospital was stark and smelled of Jeyes Fluid. Eily woke to the sound of hammering and men sailing past her with wooden planks and cans of paint. A nurse stood over her and said briskly, "We're renovating the ward, young one, so we're short on beds at the minute. But don't worry, we'll find you a place."

And so Eily was carted off on a trolley, slid into the lift, and up two stories, where she was deposited into a cot, next to a man in a bed.

"Peader, meet Eily. She's just had her appendix out."

"Well, young Eily, I'm delighted to make your acquaintance."

"I have a dog," Eily shared with the man. "Well, he's not mine, really, but he's lovely and he'll be missing me now. I have to get better soon."

She sighed at the man with teeth the color of sunshine. She was stiff and sore and her legs were scrunched up against the wooden frame but the man was hacking and spitting up red flecks and she forgot all about her worries.

Peader watched her for a while and finally he spoke. "Why don't you crawl in here beside me, Eily, and we can play Dominoes?"

Eily was glad to be out of her cage and she sat on the edge of the man's bed, watching the dominoes spill outwards like a Chinese fan.

"If you want, you can sleep here too. I'll put you where my guardian angel would be," as he made all the room in the world for her.

And so the pair slept soundly, two creatures in a single bed, until the nurses came with the breakfast trays in the morning and plucked Eily up in the air and back into her cot.

When her mother came in to see her, all Eily wanted to know was how was Banjo. "Does he miss me?"

At first, her mother sighed and nodded, but each day that passed, Eily would pose the same question and her mother would just click her teeth like she had a toothache.

"Give him my love!" she'd shout after her mother. "Tell him it won't be long now."

"Peader, did you ever have a dog?" Eily asked after her mother had left.

"I didn't, girl, no."

"Well, did you ever have something you loved more than anything in the whole wide world?"

"There was a woman once…"

"Yeah? Did she make your heart sing like Banjo does mine?"

"Well not exactly, Eily," Peader scratched his head. "But she was the closest I came to that kind of love."

"Is she gone now?"

"Ah, she's long gone, child. But it was good while it lasted."

Peader directed traffic on O'Connell Street. He wore a uniform just like the Gardaí and he was allowed to stop cars and then with a wave of his arms, let them move on. Without him helping, he said, it would be a circus out there. Eily thought of the dodgems crashing into each other at a fair. She imagined him in long white gloves, his arms dancing in elegant waves, and all the people having to heed him.

"Only I'd give it all up for love, I would," he coughed hard and a river of phlegm came out his mouth. He wiped it up with a hanky. His breath was fast and heavy. Eily was worried but she said, "Well, I love Banjo more than anything and guess what, I love you the very same."

Peader smiled weakly. "That's my girl."

Eily wished The Face would beam at her new friend and console him too but instead she put her arm around his shoulder as far as it would go and Peader slowly melted into her embrace.

Two days later, her mother and father arrived. "We're taking you home now, Eily. Your mother'll pack up your things. The car's waiting outside."

"Yippee!" Eily leaped out of her cot, even though it hurt her tummy. "I'm going home to Banjo! Banjo! Banjo!"

"Come along now, Eily," her mother was moving briskly. "Let me get this dress on you."

"Did you tell him I'm coming, did you?"

Her mother only whisked Eily's nightie off her and buttoned up the back of her blue dress.

"Oh Peader," Eily sighed. "I'll miss you terrible but I hope you get better soon and I'll come to see you in O'Connell Street, okay?"

Peader nodded and Eily could tell he was sad to see her go but she could hardly contain her delight at seeing Banjo again.

"I will, Peader, I will. Won't we, Mum, go and see Peader on his job?"

"We will indeed." Eily's mother extended her hand to Peader. "And thank you so much for taking such good care of the girl."

"A pleasure, missus, a true pleasure."

All the way home, Eily danced up and down in the back seat, singing.

"D'ye think Banjo missed me? Did he run away again? What d'ye think he'll do when he sees me?"

On and on she went, ignoring the strange feeling in her chest.

"Ban-jo, king of my so-ul!"

"Eily!" Her father's voice thundered through the car. "Banjo is gone!"

"Gone? Where?"

Her mother was wiping her face with a hanky.

"What d'you mean, Daddy, gone?"

"He was chasing the sheep at the end of the road and Colonel Timmons complained to us, said he'd call the police. We had to put him down."

"Put him down where?" Eily couldn't understand anything. Her head was on fire. All she could do was repeat what she heard.

"Dead, Eily. Banjo is dead. He was a menace to the neighborhood."

"No! No! No! It can't be," Tears gushed out of Eily's eyes, her body shivering. "Nooooo!"

"He's dead and that's that. Calm yourself, would you?"

Eily's mother turned in her seat and put her hand on Eily's shaking shoulder. "I am so sorry, dear. We had no choice."

"None at all!" Her father said.

Eily folded into a ball in the back seat, howling. There was nothing, absolutely nothing, that could fill the hollow inside her. Maybe she was being punished for stealing that cabbage last year but she'd only intended it as a gift. No matter how she tried to make sense of Banjo, her loyal companion, no longer breathing, she just couldn't.

As soon as the car pulled up at the gate, Eily shoved open the door and without saying a word, she ran all the way up to Colonel Timmons' house, a stitch in her stomach not stopping her. She banged hard on the door.

Mrs. Timmons came out, wiping her hands on her apron. "Well, I'll be..." She looked down at the girl before her.

"How *dare* you complain about Banjo! He wouldn't hurt a spider. How absolutely *dare* you!" Eily couldn't think, only let the wild fire inside her rage itself free.

"Miss, I'm sorry but..."

"But what? You took the most innocent creature, my best friend, my on-ly friend, away from me because of your... your..." and Eily could feel the word rising in her, the forbidden word she'd heard Liam use, "your *fucking* sheep!"

The look of horror on Mrs. Timmons' face made clear to Eily the power of a single word. She felt a wave of satisfaction even as the woman called her a disgrace and slammed the door on her.

Even with the wild rose bush in bloom and enough sunshine to cast shadows, the back garden was a desert to Eily. No paws scribbling all over her body any more, no wet tongue tingling her legs. No one waiting for her at the gate when she came home from the shops. Even Jim had been let go now that the weeding was finished. Only one flicker of hope remained.

Eily implored her mother to take her to O'Connell Street so she could see Peader in action. But there was never enough time. Months went by and still they didn't go. Eily wished she'd gotten Peader's address so she could write to him. When they did eventually take a bus into town, they watched him from the corner of Henry Street. Eily wanted to wave but her mother said it would be a distraction and led her towards the G.P.O., though they'd no letters to post.

"Peader!" Eily shouted as loudly as she could anyway. "It's me, your pal, Eily!"

She thought she saw him look their way for a second but there were cars stopped in the middle of the crossing and he had to shift his attention there.

Next time they ventured into town, they found traffic lights where Peader would have stood. Tall black poles with red and green lights in them. They changed color, telling motorists whether to brake or go. They looked pretty, Eily thought, like Christmas lights but they couldn't compare to her friend.

"I wonder what happened to Peader. D'ye think he lost his job?"

"Probably so," her mother said. "That's progress for you."

Several months later, her father spread The Irish Press on the table. "Lookit!" He said. "There's an article here on the changing times. Isn't that the lad was in hospital with you, Eily?"

Eily looked at the picture. "Peader my pal! Oh, he looks so smart in his uniform. I just knew he was famous!"

Eily read the caption beneath. *Peader O'Sullibhean, Dublin's last traffic coordinator, died on July 7, following a long illness.*

She stared at the photograph, watching it blur as tears dripped onto the paper until all she could see was mist. Then she crumpled it in her fist and blew kisses as she threw it in the dustbin.

EAMON

He hated the land there, people saw beauty in the lambs in the field and the sea waves below the hill, but he knew the earth was scarred long ago, the bones of the past still fighting for breath like weeds no one would pluck. The smell of the cattle in the shed made him sick.

They sang hymns in the car all the way from Dublin. *Hail Glorious Saint Patrick,* Dear Saint of our Isle. Eily and Liam in the back seat, grumbling, taking up the tune here and there and then falling silent.

"Are we near the bump yet, Daddy?"

"Not far now, girl."

"Oh good!"

They were long past Balbriggan, and once they got through Drogheda, they'd smell the seaweed, they'd be inching in to that infested place.

The bump was a hitch in the road, a swelling like a small hillock but steep enough that you'd lie down in the back and your tummy would start swirling. The girl liked it, a sensation between excitement and dread, he wasn't sure. But she seemed to live for it on these long, exhausting drives.

"Will Grandma in Port be well enough to be out of bed, d'you think?" Eily leaned into the front seat.

"We'll have to see when we get there, won't we?"

Liam was sullen, breathing these long sighs that carried the weight of the world in them. Eamon wished he'd shut up. He could hear his son chewing gum so loud, it made his ears burn.

And that monster of a headache, his head ready to explode. "Pipe down back there!" He roared at the pair behind him, though he felt badly, they had no idea the torture he was going through, his head too stuffed full of worries – he hadn't paid the milk man for weeks, the wife forever racing off to look after her mother, the abortion rights campaigners doing his head in – and not an end in sight.

Clouds the color of coal hung low over the farmhouse as they approached. The sun was in hiding. There'd be a deluge before the day was out, he was certain of that, and not even a hint of a rainbow. And wouldn't you know it, Rusty, the mangy old mutt, barking his head off at the open gate.

"Shut yer screeching for a minute, would you?" Eamon bawled at the dog, leaning out the car door for a stone to flick at him. The dog took off for the hay shed.

"Ah, they're here, Mammy, they're finally here!" Lily stopped dredging water out of the red tank and shuffled towards them.

"Well, aren't you the big girl now, young Eily? Nearly as tall as your mother! And Liam, I'd hardly know you at all."

"Ma's away with Grandma in England," Eily hooshed herself out the back door of the car and threw her arms around her aunt, resting the side of her face against her aunt's apron.

"Away with you now, girl. Sure I'm filthy. Make sure and wash yourself so you're not a mess for your granny. Go in there and say hello, why don't you? She's by the fire."

Eily ran inside, Liam slouching behind her, and Lily close behind. "I'll throw the kettle on for youse. And I'm only after opening the apply jelly…"

Eamon drove slowly over the mess of stones and parked by the field.

He couldn't help but look across the tall stalks hammered by the wind. And the well his mother had fallen into as a girl. He shivered, though it wasn't the cold.

That field.

He slept in the back room, tossing from one side to the other. He wasn't sure was it being back here again, but a gray film loomed over him. After hours staring at nothing, he went to the bathroom cabinet and helped himself to Lily's sleeping tablets.

But it wasn't an easy rest. He was being carried back to the field again, on his knees playing with the caterpillars in the grass. Only he wasn't a young boy any more but a grown man on his knees, engrossed in the earth, who knows why. And then the rustle behind him and his trousers ripped asunder and a huge thick lever thrust into his behind. And a man's groaning all over again and the terror on him when he woke up in the dark, sweat streaking off him.

You black bastard, Jack, get away from me once and for all. He was upright in bed, yelling, and not a single sound came out. *I'll show you, so I will....* His boy fist raised in anger but Jack was long gone from here, his secret taken with him, and all Eamon could do was lie back on the bed and let his breath catch up with him.

EILY

He was like the weather, her father, one minute all sullen clouds, and the next, the sun would burst through. For now, he was in a good mood. She could tell by the way he told joke after joke, slapping her knee with each punch line. He usually got all serious and made everyone pray more when her mother was away in England. He'd say, "Sure, what's she crossing the Channel for when she's got a family to feed at home?" But today, he'd been happy, pulling out the vacuum and saying, "Eily, d'ye know that me and nature have a lot in common?"

"How's that, Daddy?"

"Well, nature abhors a vacuum and to be honest," and here he sighed, pausing for effect, "so do I."

Even when she was washing the dishes after tea and handing him the plates to dry, he'd hand the odd one back, saying, "Reject!"

And she'd scrub it again, laughing. When he'd polished the shoes and lined them up like soldiers in the breakfast room, he called to her in the kitchen, "Eily, if you like the service here, tell others. If you don't, tell us!"

He had that sparkle back in his hazel eyes. It had been so long since she'd seen it through the smoke of his sadnesses.

"You'll never guess," he smiled into the mirror, combing back his silvering hair. "Uncle Jack's not well at all. In fact, an ambulance took him into the Mater this morning."

"Janey mac! What's wrong with him?"

"His heart, Eily."

"But you seem so, well, chipper."

Her father stood upright, his face more serious. "Ah sure, he's finally getting the treatment he's long needed, Eily, and I'm glad for that."

Though she was sorry to hear anyone's heart was hurting, Eily saw her chance. "Daddy... would you ever tell us a story?"

She loved her father's wild imaginings. He had a way with words. Once he'd helped her write an essay for school. "The trees wafted emerald and azure in the dawning day." She thought it sounded nice and copied it into her jotter, writing the rest herself with the help of a dictionary. She looked up every word she could find for 'green.' *Jade, turquoise, verdant.* She swirled the words around on her tongue. It gave her such pleasure, how you could make magic out of black marks on a page until they turned into light. She thought it strange how people made sharp coals out of words when they spoke as if they'd forgotten the light that had borne them. Next day, Sister Carmelita dragged her up to the front of the class and chided her for "appropriating material from elsewhere." No matter how she struggled to explain that her father had only written a single line of the two page essay, she was ignored.

"A hundred lines for you, young girl, tonight. 'I will not plagiarize the words of others.'"

When Eily asked if she could reword it to 'others' words' in order to save herself a lot of writing, Sister Carmelita pulled out the chipped ruler from her desk and whittled the roof of Eily's hands to raw skin.

"Well, let me see," Eily's father sat back in the faded rocking chair. The legs were loose and the fabric was torn on the back but her father didn't seem to have a care in the world.

"I'll tell you about Jomulduhoko."

"Who?"

"Don't you know Jomulduhoko? Surely everyone's heard of him. He was a sad man, a lonely man." Her father settled into his chair and closed his eyes, arms crossed at his chest as if he were reminiscing about something that happened a long time ago.

"He was a laborer, our Jo, come up from the country, didn't know a soul in the entire city of Dublin."

"Not one?"

"Not a single one, Eily. And poor man, he had a mess of a time trying to find employment. No one would hire him, you see, because he had only the one shirt to his name. It used to be white but he'd worn it so much, it had turned almost gray."

Eily sighed, wondering why he didn't go to The Legion of Mary or St. Vincent de Paul for help.

"So he went into Miss Doyle's shop."

"Oh, he lived locally, did he?"

"He did indeed, Eily. Somewhere around though no one knew exactly where he laid his head at night. So as I was saying, into Miss Doyle's he went and he looked around at the rows of jars on the shelves, a rainbow of sweets of all colors.

"'I'll have a quarter pound of licorice All Sorts, please,' he asked Miss Doyle. 'And a half dozen Scots Clan. Oh, and give me a half pound of those Clove Drops too, will you?'

"Now Miss Doyle wasn't born yesterday, she surely wasn't, so she asked him was he new to the parish. He said indeed he was, hired to take care of Father Mulligan's garden. 'Oh,' says Miss Doyle, naturally she was impressed. No wonder he looked a bit dirty, down on his knees all day in the earth. 'Well, that explains it, then.' She smiled her best smile at him, noticing how white his teeth were, even if there weren't many of them. 'And what else can I get you?'

'A nice slice of ham'd be nifty.' Jo said. And Lord help us, while her back was turned, dropping sweets in white paper bags and weighing them on her little scale, all the while our Jo had his hand in the cash register and was slipping a few quid into his trouser pocket.

"Miss Doyle wrapped the ham in wax and slid it over the counter.

"'There you have it now, sir.' And she scribbled in her white note pad, totting up the charges."

"Wouldn't the cash register do that, Daddy?" Eily asked.

"Not in those days, no, not back then."

"How long ago was this?"

"Ah," her father opened his eyes. "I can't be exactly sure. But quite a while. It was the talk of the parish back then."

"Oh." Eily's eyebrows raised in wonder.

"Well, Jo put out his hand, his fingernails all scummy and said, as confident as you like, 'Mr. Mulduhoko! A pleasure to meet you.' He had a way about him that you'd trust him with your last tenner.

"So anyway, he says to Miss Doyle, 'Would you kindly put it on my bill and I'll pay you at the end of the week when I get paid.'

"'Oh,' says Miss Doyle, offering her hand out to shake his. 'I'd be only delighted!'

"And so she pulled out her packet of invoices and wrote one up for Mr. Mulduhoko. On Friday, there was no sign of him, though. Nor on Saturday. Nor even Sunday. Miss Doyle thought he must be busy helping Father Mulligan get ready for Mass.

"It was lashing hard on the Tuesday when Jo finally walked into the shop again, dripping wet he was. 'Ah, Mr. Mulduhoko. I'm glad to see you. Will you be paying off your bill today?'

"'Ah no, Miss Doyle, I'm sorry but the priest, God help him, says it'll be month's end before he can pay me.'

"'I see.' Miss Doyle let out a long sigh. 'Well, it can't be helped. I'll just have to wait.'

"'Thank you, Miss Doyle.' Our Jo was all polite and gushing. 'Now, could you get me a sliced pan and a half pint of raspberry ripple ice cream?'

"Miss Doyle slid open the ice cooler and no sooner had she turned than he had his hand in the till again."

"My God, didn't she hear him at all?" Eily was enthralled.

"Not at all. Didn't you know Miss Doyle is deaf in one ear and she doesn't hear too well out of the other either?

"So this went on week after week. Every time Jo came in, sure, he'd have another brilliant excuse handy. And week after week, Miss Doyle'd make all sorts of noises but what could she do? Sure, he was a servant of God, how could she turn him away?

"Well, it wasn't until her sister, Evelyn, came to visit, that things got serious. There were no flies on Evelyn, not a single one. And she peered into the till through her thick black rimmed glasses and said, 'I believe you're short here, sister.'"

"She called her sister?"

"Indeed she did. No one has ever known Miss Doyle's first name. I couldn't tell you if she ever had one at all. But oh, her sister smelled a rat. Well, who should come strolling in through the door only himself, all big-eyed and smiling, and asking for a cut of the best lamb they had.

"'I apologize,' said Evelyn, 'but we can't be giving you any more items until you pay off your bill, which, I might add, is substantial.'

"'I'll be in with a check tomorrow, I promise. Things have been a bit pinched lately, what with my dying mother in Carlow and my two sisters without a job between them. What's a man to do with so many to take care of besides himself?' And he looked so forlorn standing there, his shoulders all slumped, that Miss Doyle was about to take pity on him yet again.

"Only this time, her sister piped in. She wouldn't hear of it. 'Well, sir, you come in here tomorrow with your check and we'll give you the lamb then. All right?'

"Now she had one of those voices that you'd call imperious…"

"What does that mean?" Eily asked, though she didn't want him to stop talking.

"Scary, Eily, scary." Her father yawned, long and drawling. He was getting weary, she could tell. It was long past her bedtime.

"So what happened then? Did he bring his check like he said?"

"He did, poor man. But sure, it was a bad check. He hadn't a farthing in his pocket nor even his bank account.

"Well, once he had the lamb in hand, he scarpered out the door and the Miss Doyles went trotting off to the Bank of Ireland the very next morning. But sure, there wasn't a bean to be gleaned from this check. And Miss Doyle threw her arms up in frustration.

"'We'll have to contact the police, sister.' Evelyn said with authority. 'I'm going down to the Garda station right now!'

"And off she marched, all the way down Old Finglas Road until she got where she was going. She filed a claim against Jomulduhoko and it wasn't long before the guards were banging on the door of his little cottage."

"How did they know where he lived?"

"Sure, it was on the check, wasn't it? Well, poor Jo, he knew his handy number was up. He bolted the front and back doors and put all the furniture he could find up against both entrances. He already had the venetian blinds drawn and he hid in the box room, hunkered down on the floor, shivering with dread."

"Did the guards get through the door?"

"Sure, they probably did eventually, though I don't rightly recall. I heard someone tell how he escaped out onto the roof and clung there to the thatch, hanging over the awning all night long. And at first light, when the guards had given up and gone home, he leaped down onto the ground, probably cracking a rib or two and hobbled off into the day, never to be seen again."

"Oh," Eily was glad somehow that he got away. She knew what it was like to be locked in a dark room, even if you did it to yourself. If she'd gotten pocket money like some girls in school, she'd have given it to him. What kind of life was that, having to lie and steal to keep bread in your mouth? But she said nothing, only sent him a rose from her heart to keep him going, wherever he was now.

"And more's the pity for Miss Doyle. She was out of pocket so much, she had to close down the shop for a while and when she opened again, she stopped selling meat of any kind. She was never the same again, she looked ashen, like someone had shaken her too long and taken the wind out of her."

"Oh Daddy, I wish the story had a happy ending, though in a way, I suppose it does." And she pulled down the hot water bottles from their hooks, the wild doings of Jomulduhoko floating through her head. Even the kettle boiling couldn't rouse her father from his chair. She'd sleep well tonight.

EAMON

It irritated him to see all the old dossers hanging around outside Gogan's after the 12 o'clock. Just waiting to get their paws on a pint. Sure, probably most of them hadn't even been to Mass at all and they standing around in gaggles, whinging about being on the dole.

Every week, someone or other would stop him on his way home and offer to buy him a drink. He was proud he'd taken the Pledge, vowing to God and himself never to let a sip of alcohol pass beyond his lips again. He'd done it enough in his rugby days, the lads passing pints around like water after a win, all guff and bluster. He'd never really taken to it, the sharp tang of warm liquid that made your head spin and had you saying things you'd wish you hadn't in the morning. But he went along, just the same.

Dempsey, it was, said he was a lightweight, never mind he was a second row forward, and challenged him to a drinking duel at the Irish Rugby Banquet in Wynn's Hotel. He couldn't refuse, with the whole team, even the manager, egging him on. Must have had a dozen lagers, one after the other, until Dempsey blurred into the mist. It plagued him the whole drive home that Dempsey had won the bet. Bloody bastard, sure, he was all talk and twice his size to begin with. He'd more room to hold his liquor. But no one mentioned that, only gave him a rousing for losing.

Only hours before, some young lad had chased him down Abbey Street, mad for an autograph. And what had he gotten from the day but a blinding headache and the wife unable to drive. He was fuming as they left O'Connell Street, the road a winding riddle before him. And she going on and on about the curse of drinking or something.

Why had she moved to put her hand on his cheek, anyway? He knew how to drive, he knew that much at least. But on she went blathering and what could he do but raise his arm to block hers, who knows what she was up to, only he didn't gauge the distance right. Crack! his arm went against her cheek and she screaming at him to pull over NOW! Her face swelling like a red balloon and blood around her eye.

He didn't want to think about it but there it was: the image of her slowly hooshing herself out of the car and walking off into the dark and he having to get himself home in one piece.

She'd been gone a week and he with no iota of where she was. The children pulling on him for food, for answers. And then she rang. His heart skipped a beat when he heard her voice again. It seemed to be coming from another planet.

"I've been staying with Uncle Er," she said slowly, in that deliberate English voice of hers. "He said, 'if you go back to him, you'll have sealed your fate.' But we have children, Eamon, that need taking care of. Can you do it alone?"

It was then he decided the Pledge was the only answer. He didn't want Brother Ernest badmouthing him as well. Sure, he could hardly take care of himself.

She'd come back, her face still raw under the make up and she told the crying girl she'd been in an accident but was all right now.

Yes, he'd done the right thing, forsaking the booze. *Uisce beatha,* they called whiskey, the water of life. Death, more like, he mused as old McTaggart from Finglas raised his cap to him and said, "Can I buy you a Guinness, Eamon? They'll be opening any minute."

Sick of it, he was, these bowsies wasting money they didn't have on rubbish.

Then a wondrous idea floated into his head. He could feel his heart lift up as he moved towards the man with his cap in his hand.

"No, thanks very much, Mikey." He was almost gleeful now. "I won't have a drink with you but I'd be delighted to take the money instead."

McTaggart swiped his cap across his forehead, the look on his face more than enough reward for Eamon as he sauntered past, leaving a crew of black crows staring after him.

EILY

Miss Patterson shoved Eily into the queue.

"Get that hair out of your eyes, child," she said. Eily could feel the kindness under her gruff words.

"Do we *have* to have our pictures taken, Miss?"

"Yes, you do. Each of you girls. Then you'll take it home to your parents and they can purchase it for you."

"But what if they don't want to?" Mary O'Gorman asked.

"They will. Now stand up straight while you're waiting. And take deep breaths – it will put some color in your faces."

Eily held the wet photograph with the edges of her fingers. The girl that looked out at her seemed pale. Did she really look like that? Half bewildered, half baffled at the flashing bulb that made her eyes blink. Her navy head band was pulled way back on her head and her dicky bow was askew. If she squinted, she could see traces of that brightness that used to fill her whole being. It was a bit dimmed all right, like the tail end of a rainbow on a cloudy day.

Her mother took one look at it and went back to pouring flour out of a sieve onto the cutting board. "I'm making treacle tart today for pudding. You'll enjoy that."

"What about the picture?"

"No, we'll not be buying it."

"But why? There's no pictures of me in the entire house."

"We're not buying it, and that's that."

"But Mum, all the girls…"

"No, Eileen, no. We have to look at you enough as it is."

Eily left the photo on the table and went out to sit on the front stoop. The red paint cracked and peeled in the heat and sometimes left a stain on her clothes. She propped her elbows on her legs and her palms under her chin. A boy walked up the drive of Mahon's house across the road. They were the only Protestants in the parish and they kept to themselves. Eily had heard that they were moving to Oregon in America. She'd seen pictures in school of the tall, emerald green trees and huge mountains. She imagined the family packing their suitcases and flying off on a jet to a better home where they could start again, make new friends, people who wouldn't judge them, who'd open their hearts and say, *Welcome.* It was what her own heart longed to do but no one was interested.

Softly, she sang to herself, *Somewhere ov-er the rainbow, there's a land I heard of once in a lull-a-by…* She imagined a rainbow arcing across the heavens from Mahon's all the way to Oregon and a giant pot of gold treasures waiting to greet them. She wished she could follow the trail, fly off somewhere warm and gentle, a place where she'd be greeted with wide open arms. It softened the sadness floating inside her. Some fine day, she'd find a path out of this world where she seemed always to be a stranger.

Oh, they were in such a lather on the day itself. Almost eight years she'd been waiting. The Big Day, her father called it, when she'd be marrying the True Prince of Heaven. But Eily was not a happy bride. She had begged her mother to buy her the silk dress, a froth of slinky folds she could drizzle her fingers along. Soft and creamy when it caught the light, it seemed to shimmer. Eily was in love. But her mother insisted on the starched cotton dress, all hard, gunned with little holes throughout which was supposed to make it more attractive, the sales lady said. It cost three pounds less.

"You'll get more wear out of this one," Eily's mother assured her. "You know how messy you are with food." The silk would be ruined before she knew it.

Her veil was a crusty organza and it felt stiff as a corpse to Eily. She implored her mother to make ringlets of her hair, like she'd seen the fancy Irish dancers do. Maybe her mother would want a picture of her if she looked like other girls. She knew they wound tresses in wet rags overnight to form tight curls of their hair. Her mother had no idea how to do it, being unaccustomed to Irish ways, but she made an effort to wind Eily's russet locks around a half dozen scrawny curlers.

On the morning itself, her mother yanked and tugged at her hair but the curlers wouldn't budge. She cried out as her mother tried to unleash the wire cylinders, hairs catching and ripping away from her scalp.

"Heaven help us," Eily's mother said, unearthing the black clips, but the curlers seemed determined to stay.

"Janey Mac!" her father roared when he came into the kitchen, and saw Eily's red eyes and her mother making mince meat of her hair. "We're going to be late for Mass. Today of all days!"

He circled the pair once, twice, eyeing up the gravity of the situation.

"Just cut her hair off now, Mother! We can't be late." And he made a lunge for the drawer with the scissors in it. "If you don't, I will."

Eily's mother raced into the breakfast room, grabbed a coat from the rack where clothes were airing, threw it over Eily's head and pushed her out the back door.

"We'll see you there, Eamon. Don't worry. We'll be on time."

And the pair huddled under an umbrella, pushing into the wind, as they trudged down the avenue, taking the short cut through Cremore, past her school, and down the Washerwoman's Hill, until they got to Bill's Barber Shop, across the road from the church.

Eily's mother shoved her inside the door. The windows were all steamy as if they were crying.

"I can't do a thing with her hair. And she's making her First Holy Communion at ten o'clock this morning."

Before she knew it, the barber had her in a big leather chair and he worked his magic, unraveling the mess on Eily's scalp, so much more gently than her mother.

One look in the mirror and tears sprung to Eily's eyes. Her hair was a wiggle of tight bedsprings, nothing like the young girls who danced.

"Well, at least you won't be taking your vows, lovie, with a head full of curlers and clips. Now that wouldn't do at all, would it?"

Eily shook her head, glad to see the curlers resigned to the dustbin. The barber slipped half a crown into her palm as she left and Eily let it slide in the sweat of her palm as she crossed the road towards Our Lady of Dolours and her waiting father.

The organ was bleating out a long, sonorous tune as the young girls floated down the aisle in a sea of virgin white.

But Eily's consolation prize could not be taken away from her. She had managed to talk her mother into buying her a pair of satin underpants. Cheaper than a dress, and she could enjoy the warm slink on her thighs. It would be her secret.

As was customary, after the service, she went door to door on the road, to show the neighbors her outfit and be given a slice of cake or a shilling. She filled her beaded bag with coins and chewed on some icing from an old fruit cake Mrs. Gallagher handed her. She felt ashamed of her stiff dress, her tattered Mary Janes. She longed to show off her precious under garment, to let everyone see the real beauty.

Finally, at Costello's, she couldn't help herself – up came the skirt of her dress in one swoosh.

"Look, Mrs. Costello. My dress may not be much but see what I have hidden here." Mrs. Costello looked away, embarrassed and almost shut the door on her as she gave her a few pennies. Eily didn't care. Her skin felt all tingly.

Mr. Burke was not at all put off by her rash display. He invited her in, roughly, by the arm. "C'mere," he said, tossing the cigarette from his mouth, "give us those knickers."

There was a commotion behind the door, its leaded glass

echoing every move like a taunting teacher. It happened so quickly, Eily could hardly take it in, a minute or an hour, she wasn't sure, all rough and tussle, and then a pool of smear dripping down her right leg, as Mr. Burke opened the front door again and pushed her outside.

Eily took the new cotton hankie from her bag and wiped herself down. Her pants were a gloppy mess. She'd have to wash them in the upstairs sink. If she said a word, they'd say it was all her fault and maybe it was. Why did she have to show off like that? Wasn't that her mother's job, to be admired? She bit her tongue hard as she slid out of the damp pants, settling them in her purse under the sixpences and half crowns. If anyone knew, she might be shoved under the stairs again, or even worse, locked into the freezing outside loo, spiders slinking over the toilet lid. And holy mother, what if it was the coal house for her? Soiled even on her wedding day.

When she got home, she went straight upstairs and buried her pants in the back of the wardrobe. She counted out her earnings, almost two guineas. Sliding her bag under the bed, she pulled out her jotter, scribbling, *Girls who don't hide their light under a bushel get themselves into too much trouble,* a tear for every word.

Now that Eily was married to God, she was required to go to Mass every Sunday. Her father would take her by the hand and sit her next to him in the front pew. He said it was a sin to be late for Mass and so they always arrived a half hour early. When she knelt and closed her eyes, she'd see a garden, not like O'Reilly's or any other she'd laid eyes on but a wild field without beginning or end and it overflowing with foliage of all shapes, swaying to their special tune. The sun was a kind of spinning halo in the sky. Every strand of grass brimming with silvery light you couldn't put a name on. It was her true home, she knew, and she'd see herself dancing there, a young girl, pure as the petals streaming down her hair and she lit up from inside with a happiness she may never know in this life.

She wondered why her father had to pray so much, lines spilling out like a long, boring invoice. God didn't need all those words, he was happy with silence. All he wanted was for your heart to be glad. He understood the language of the heart, for hadn't he forged it himself? It was so far beyond words recited like a robot. He'd let you go on and on with your hymns and your Creeds and Our Fathers but a simple burst of love in your chest gave him such joy, Eily was convinced.

Sometimes when Father Lamb was droning on about confessing your sins, Eily would pick the prettiest flower from the vase on the altar, hopefully a rose – God loved roses – and she'd imagine tossing it up to the heavens and it landing bull's eye on his lap. How could people sin when they were conjured of pure light? It wasn't any wonder they called the decades of the Rosary mysteries. There was so much she just didn't understand of this world.

Still, she prayed with the rest of the parishioners. She'd do anything to make her father happy. But she wasn't sure he was, or not for long. He could crack a good joke, slapping his strong hand on your knee at the punch line and they'd share a laugh together. But then he'd sink back into that dark silence again. Even when he hardly muttered a word for days, she knew he wasn't quiet inside. There was a tornado brewing in that wild head of his and she longed with all her heart to calm it.

He didn't even seem pleased when he'd come at her in the bedroom. Something would release from him for a few minutes but then he'd zip up his trousers and that something would tighten even more.

So she got down on her knees and prayed. It saddened her sitting next to him at Mass, and he sing-songing his prayers so loudly, she knew the whole church could hear him, and maybe people out on the street too. He didn't even keep time with the others, only wired to his own moon, he was.

During the sermon, Eily sat on the hard wooden bench and let her eyes wander round the windows, looking for that special gleam that told her an angel was nearby. At communion, she'd watch the people queue up along the middle aisle towards the priest, heads bowed. She had to squint her eyes to find the light inside each person. Sometimes an old man would be so hunched and in pain, she couldn't find it. It hurt her heart to feel the cowl of darkness around him so she'd blow him a secret kiss or plant a chirping bird on his shoulder. Although she was only half dreaming, she'd be amazed to see the man stand a little taller, a little more juice in his step.

It was her mother opened the first letter. Eily came home from school to find her sitting on the kitchen stool staring at the wall. A sheet of paper lay on her lap. She was still in her dressing gown though it was almost time for dinner. Yellow soup bubbled in the pan.

"Ma...?"

Eily knew something was wrong when her mother didn't correct her for being 'common.' She wouldn't let anyone watch Tolka Row, even though it had been filmed at the bottom of the Washerwoman's Hill and named after their local river. "Picking up a Dublin accent will be the end of you," she'd say. "No one will hire you anywhere."

Eily wondered why jobs were important when she was only eight and a half.

An envelope sat on the table. The address was written in big, cursive letters scrawled to the right. Though Eily adored reading, she could hardly make out the words. It had a Dublin postmark.

"Is it another bill, Mum?" She asked softly.

Her mother didn't move for a minute, then turned her face towards Eily. Her cheeks were damp. "It's your father," she said quietly, looking into the distance. "I knew I'd rue the day he asked me to marry him..."

Eily had heard the story many times, how her mother had been nursing in England and went to a dance one night. There was a rugby crowd over from Ireland. She caught sight of a handsome man in an oversized suit with lapels that made him look like a gangster. She had her eye on him all evening and oh magic, he started walking in her direction, his eyes twinkling, but stopped just before he reached her. He'd asked her friend to dance. Her mother had been taken aback but pushed down her disappointment, the way she always did. Then, as the music slowed, he approached her again and this time took her hand and led her out on the floor.

Eily always liked that part, her father's mahogany curls lilting round his face, his arms swaddling her mother, maybe the beginnings of her in that embrace. They agreed to meet the next day in the park. It was November, a mist hovering over the swollen apples. They picked pine cones up off the ground and tossed them into the hedgerow.

They wrote letters back and forth and eventually her mother took the B&I across the sea. She met the rugby team and the captain said, "So you're the fog that delayed him."

Her mother was not welcomed by her father's family, not at all. His own mother, a wide-hipped farm woman, declared, "If you want to marry my son, you better become a Catholic." And so she did, though she never took to all the formality and long-winded prayers.

And then on Dun Laoghaire pier one sharp night, they strolled arm in arm towards the lighthouse. When they were on the edge of the point, he turned to face her and asked her if she'd be his bride.

"A long shiver went through me," her mother had told her many's the time. "I knew it would be a hard road but what else could I do?"

She, who had left a man weeping at the station in Yorkshire as her train chugged away because she found out his parents were deaf and dumb, and she just wouldn't have children handicapped like that.

Always practical, her mother, in every way and yet there she was helpless but to follow her heart, no matter the murmurings of her mind.

"What about Daddy?"

"An anonymous letter complaining that he prays so loudly at Mass."

"Oh," Eily sighed. She remembered Mark Ryan jeering her before the May Day Procession, asking if her father needed a tannoy so he'd be heard in the crowd.

"What do they say?"

"They're threatening him, Eily, threatening us. It's an irritation to people. Why oh why can't he pray like everyone else?"

"Because he's not like anyone else, Mum," she said, her heart torn between her mother's grief and her father's need.

"If they'd only signed it, then I'd go and speak to them, try to explain he's not well. It's an illness…"

"It is not! Daddy is fine. He just wants to get God's ear before anyone else." But she wasn't sure that was true. It embarrassed her to hear him chanting his prayers from inside when she was walking up the church steps. They were all outsiders, she thought, what with her father's strange ways, her mother's foreign accent, and herself who saw light and faces not of this world. They were like three paper airplanes hovering in space, belonging to no one.

"I'm sorry, Mum," she tried. "If I got my hands on that person, I'd wring their neck so I would!"

"You have to understand, Eily, that people have different needs. I can accept someone being upset but I do wish they'd let us know who they were."

Eily lunged for the paper hankies and handed her mother one. She didn't reach out to take it and it landed like a lost feather on her lap.

"I'd better take that soup off the stove. Goodness, it's almost one o'clock. What was I thinking?" Her mother stood, brushing Eily aside and went about her business as if the world was as perfect as she usually pretended it was.

Whenever Uncle Jack came to visit, he'd bring a box of Cadbury's Contrast and place them in Eily's hand. He wasn't really her uncle, but her father's uncle. He seemed lonely to Eily. He lived in a flat on the Rathgar road in Dublin, with no wife or family. Her father said he preferred his own company. And he was quiet, to be sure, only speaking when someone addressed him. It made Eily nervous watching her father pace the room like a snared animal, stopping only to refill his uncle's tea. He called him only, "Jack," and if it weren't for Eily, the room would be silent as a coffin.

Ever since he'd been in hospital for his weak heart, Uncle Jack would hand the girl her present and shuffle into the rocking chair by the hearth. Eily could feel the heaviness lurking around his shoulders and she'd make a big fuss of the chocolates, though she preferred sandwiches to sweets.

For his sake, she'd pretend to dive after her favorites, but always offer him first choice. Mostly, she enjoyed emptying the box and turning the wax holder upside down so it looked like a typewriter. And she'd go outside and sit against the apple tree, typing out the letters she imagined would be on the toffee swirls or the rich raspberry.

> *Dear God,*
>
> *I wish you were here next to me, so we could sit together and enjoy the clouds. I miss you. If you come, you can have any of the chocolates that are left, except for the coconut cream, because Daddy favors that one and he's only allowed one sweet a day with his diabetes. Write back soon, will you? Your friend, Eily. P.S. I don't like asking you for too much but would you ever let us know who's sending those letters about Da praying too loud? Ma's having a terrible time over it. Thanks a million.*

Uncle Jack had made all his money on boxing and Eily's father said they'd be rich some day, for he had promised to leave everything to his nephew in his will. They had an arrangement. Eily couldn't imagine what rich really meant. The wild rose that struggled to flower by the back wall and the blackberry thickets behind Miss Doyle's shop were her riches. She couldn't think of a thing she might buy, maybe a Choc Ice on a warm summer day, but how often did that happen? Well, maybe some books, she loved to read. Enid Blyton was her hero. She'd already lapped up *You're A Good Friend, Noddy!* and all of the *Four Marys* series from the library.

She still thrilled at the memory of her mother taking her into town to buy a new suit for her father. "He's up for promotion," she'd told Eily. It was raining hard and they'd had to wait almost an hour for the bus. By the time they got to O'Connell Street, it was half past five. Her mother clicked her teeth hard. "If we're to do our shopping before closing, we'll have to move quickly." She'd dropped a pound note into Eily's palm. "I want you to cross over to Eason's for me and get a box of vellum stationery. It *must* be vellum, the kind with an ink stain on it. Just ask the assistant to help you."

Eily wove a path across the road and shuffled, dripping, into Eason's. The place was brimming with new books, not the old, tattered kind she'd worn out at Drumcondra library. She ran her fingers along the wall that had a sign saying, New Novels.

She couldn't help picking up a book. The feel and smell of it made her skin tingle. And then she'd seen it. *Five Go Down to the Sea* by Enid Blyton, her favorite writer in the entire world. She lunged at it and opened the first page. Tantalizing like a ripe fruit dangling off a tree that wasn't yours, she drank in the story of five adventurers all piling into a boat. Oh God, she'd been dying to know what would happen to them but time was ticking away. She could feel a gurgle rising up in her throat. Three shillings. She sighed. She had to have it.

Her heart lurching, she'd reached up and put the box of writing paper and the book on the counter. The assistant took Eily's money, casual as you like, and put the purchases in a paper bag and the change on top. Eily wondered if it was how robbers felt when they raided a bank, the sharp crossbars in her chest.

It wasn't until they got home that her mother asked her for the stationery and change. Eily foostered in her pockets. "I might've lost it, Mum," she said at first but her mother looked so distraught, Eily couldn't lie to her.

She sat on the hearth's edge and out spilled the whole story about Enid Blyton's newest creation and how Eily couldn't, just could not help herself and how she was really sorry and she'd return it first thing in the morning.

Her mother had turned the book over and back. "And a hard-cover, if you don't mind. I don't even buy those for myself. They cost the earth!"

Eily set out next morning on foot the three miles into town. She'd save the bus fare to give to her mother as an apology. All the way down Botanic Avenue, all she could think about was how the book would turn out. She'd tried to read some in bed last night but had just got to the exciting bit when the boat gets caught in a storm when her father came in to say his usual good night.

She was dreaming up endings in her head as she walked, the book carefully placed back in its striped paper bag and that, inside her coat. She liked having the Famous Five so close to her. She thought she might have been friends with most of them, except the toffee-nosed one, if they'd been real.

It was almost lunch time by the time Eily got to O'Connell Street. She pushed her way through the milling crowds until she came to Eason's. But her heart felt heavy as concrete when she got to the entrance. Twice, she stepped inside and twice she walked back out again, the second time nearly knocking down an old lady who was hurrying in out of the rain.

Eily felt cold and tired. And she would have loved a mug of hot cocoa but she forgot about all that as she pulled the precious book out of her coat. She fondled the cover, almost kissing it, and once she decided, she felt light as a feather. She scooched herself into the farthest corner of the entrance, under the awning. Water was dripping in great plops off the fringe of it. It was striped blue and green, just like their paper bags. A bit like the ocean she longed to see, and felt it was a sign that she should stand there in the freezing cold and finish the entire book before returning it.

Her heart was beating fast at first, wondering if a Garda would come along and arrest her and then she'd really be finished. But once she got into the adventure again, she was so absorbed that time stopped. She lost all sense of where she was, or even who. On and on she turned each page, in the grip of the high seas, working hard with the Famous Five to solve the mystery of the lights flashing from the tower, even as their boat was being pushed towards the jagged rocks.

She almost shouted out loud when she realized she'd guessed the ending before she read it. She was both proud of herself and disappointed. She'd come to the final page. Here was a world where anything could happen but it always turned out right in the end.

With a sigh, she folded the book closed, tucked it into its paper pouch and was relieved to see the three shillings dropped back into her palm.

"I'm sorry, God. Well, not really," she sang to herself as she looked across at Clery's clock. It was half past three already. She pulled the hood of her gabardine tight around her face and legged it the whole way home, feeling the gaping space by her chest where the book had once been.

What was the point of fretting over money, she wondered. If she had it now, she'd get a new pair of slippers for her mother, who still wore her own mother's silk dressing gown though it was threadbare, and satin slippers that came from Africa so long ago, the colors had faded into a burnt orange. And they were never intended for the deep chill of Ireland, Eily wagered.

Why did her parents always yell at each other about bills and pennies? When Eily grew up, she promised herself she'd never waste a thought on money, like them, but earn just enough to keep her going. Besides, the angels would take care of her, she knew that much.

The phone rang just as Uncle Jack was leaving. Eily raced to answer it.

"Hello?" She always felt excited with the mouthpiece next to her ear, wondering whose voice would come tissuing out of the air. But all she heard was a kind of shuffling and a crackle before the line went dead. Eily was disappointed but she knew sometimes there'd be a wrong number. She ran out to the gate as Uncle Jack was getting into the taxi. "Cheerio now!" she smiled at him. "And thank you again for the lovely chocolates."

After he'd gone, her mother asked her who'd telephoned.

"No one."

"It can't have been no one."

"It was. Or someone who dialed the wrong number." Eily opened her arms to the glint of sun between clouds.

"Tsk!" her mother seemed worried, as if she didn't quite believe it. "Did you hear anything?"

"Just someone breathing, I suppose."

"Oh dear," her mother unlatched the front door and went back inside. "That's not good. Not good at all."

It must have been 2 a.m. when the phone ringing thundered through the house. It woke everyone. Eily rubbed the sleep from her eyes and trundled downstairs to find her mother putting the receiver back on the hook.

"Who was it, Ma?"

"That's not my name!"

"Sorry. Mum…"

"The same caller that's rung for five days now."

"But it's the middle of the night."

"I know. But she says…"

"She?"

"The woman who's upset about your father's praying."

"Her? I thought she wrote letters."

"Yes, she began that way." Her mother walked into the kitchen and put the kettle on. "But now she's ringing. She says she wants us to feel how it is for her to hear something that disturbs her."

"God! Does Daddy know?"

"He does but it's not going to change him. He wouldn't even come down to answer the phone."

"He probably just prays for her."

"He should be praying for all of us, as if it would do any good whatsoever!" Her mother poured hot water into her cup so fast, it spilled over onto the counter. Tea was the answer to all the ills of the world.

EAMON

She was in a tizzy about her mother's gold necklace. Couldn't find it anywhere. "Where could it possibly have gone? I never lose… *any*thing." Round and round like a chicken she went, looking in the dining room cabinet, all the kitchen drawers. She was giving him a headache, so she was, with her hysterics. He told her to look in her chest of drawers but no, she said, she'd looked there twenty times if she'd looked once.

"It was my father's last gift to Mother. He brought it back from Africa. I'll be distraught if it's gone." She was so tensed up, he climbed the stairs himself even though it hurt his bad leg. The diabetes was taking its toll. He emptied the drawers in her dressing table, the oak chest at the foot of her bed. Nothing but underpants and slips. He hardly saw them these days. She always wore the same flannel nightie. He draped a beige slip from his fingers like it was a dead animal, then tossed it back on top of the other carefully folded ones.

As a last try, he pulled back the counterpane and felt under the bed. His hand slammed into something hard and he drew back in surprise. He reached again and pulled out a glass bottle. For a second, he wondered if she'd been drinking on the sly though he'd not taken her for a toker. He drew his glasses out of his pocket and read the label. "COCP. Mrs. M. Massey. Must be taken continuously."

"Mother!" He marched back down to the kitchen. "Moth-er!"

"What is it, Eamon? Can't you see I'm busy here?"

"What the hell are these?" He threw the bottle on the table. That got her attention. She stopped her foostering and picked it up, shoving it in the pocket of her apron.

"Where did you find them?"

Oh, that got her, he could tell. She had a secret up her sleeve, bedad she did.

"It was your necklace I was after."

"I told you I looked in the bedroom already."

"Answer me, Mother!"

She sat down on the chair, her face all caved in. Finally, she took the bottle out of her apron and put it standing on the table.

"That..." she sighed, "is a preventative."

"For what?"

"For pregnancy..."

He scratched his head, puzzled for a minute. Then the light dawned. "You're not telling me these are.. are.. contraceptives?"

She nodded. His head was on fire. What would Father Lamb say? A roar was building in his voice. "It.. you can't... it's against the *law!*"

"Calm down, Eamon. You know as well as I do that we can't afford another..."

"Blast you, woman!" He was turning in circles, couldn't collect his thoughts in one place. "Where would you get such a thing?"

"England. I got them by prescription when I was visiting Mother."

The sweat was rolling off him, his stomach retching. "You mean to tell me you've been using... these... these... when we've been...?"

She just nodded, didn't say a word. That really got him going. He picked the bottle up, struggled upstairs again, and emptied the lot straight down the toilet. "Where they belong!"

He went into the garden to clear his head but it was exploding. *Forgive her father for she has sinned oh God so have I by association Father Lamb'll murder us we'll end up behind bars Forgive me Father* – oh, his head dizzy with lightning sparks as he fell to his knees and joined his shaking hands in prayer.

When he came back inside, she was still sitting where he'd left her. He pulled down the mug with the rosary beads in it, knelt down and said, "I'll be sleeping in the back room from now on."

He came from old money, Mr. Comerford. That's what Eily had heard, and she thought it strange a man who wore a three-piece suit and immaculate shoes could be her godfather. He came from the same village her father was raised in, Port, although he was a Protestant, and she'd not heard tell of him until now.

It was soon after her tenth birthday when he'd first arrived at the front door, a carnation in his breast pocket. His fine hair was slicked back, it had the look of grasses that had been weighted down by mud. His tie was striped purple and white, like a circus zebra. Her father took him into the dining room, where they spread out sheaves of paper and talked seriously about insurance premiums and tax-free benefits. As he was leaving, he called Eily to him, and said, "Aren't you a pretty one?" and he plucked the carnation out of his pocket and handed it to her. It was white with pink flecks on it.

"I'll be back for you, young Eily," he said, and a hint of cologne wafted into the hallway as he left.

Her father had a light in his face she'd not seen before. "His business," he said to no one in particular, "could keep us in turnips and mash for a long while."

Eily was glad to hear it especially as her father had not gotten the promotion he'd hoped for.

When Eily came home from school the next day, her father was standing at the gate waiting for her. He was shifting quickly from one foot to the other and he had a look on him that surprised Eily.

"I've grand news for you, young girl," her father raised her hand and rested it in his as they walked towards the house together. "Mr. Comerford just rang a minute ago, and you'll never believe it but he wants to be your godfather! Isn't that a blessing we weren't expecting?"

Eily wasn't sure what to think. Hardly a word had passed between them. Why would he want to be her godfather and what did that really mean? And didn't her father keep his distance from Protestants?

But her father had no time for questions. He kept saying what a boon it was, grace from Heaven. He was more excited, it seemed, than Eily was. But she was glad to see her father risen out of his black moods and so she nodded slowly, dizzily, in agreement.

Not a week had passed before Mr. Comerford appeared at the front door again. He didn't like to drive, her father had told her, so hired his own personal driver, a chauffeur, he was called. After the two men had chatted behind the closed sitting room door, Mr. Comerford asked Eily if she'd like to go for a drive to celebrate their new relations. She didn't want to but before she could speak, her father had her gingham cape around her shoulders and she was out the door. "Eamon, I'll have you drive us. Eily and I will sit in the back seat together."

His chauffeur was ushered into the living room where her mother fed him thawed barm brack from Hallowe'en and steaming tea, and off they went, around the block, past Miss Doyle's, and out past the parish, to places Eily hadn't seen before.

The car was a bright, almost gold Humber Imperial, it said on the bumper, and the seats were soft. Eily sank into the back one. In a flash, her godfather slid in next to her.

"Are you enjoying yourself, young Eily with your hair of fire?" Mr. Comerford asked.

She nodded, though she couldn't really take in the blue fields and the passing oaks, she had a funny feeling in her ribs.

Around and around they drove for what seemed like hours until somehow they came back to her road.

"Stop here, Eamon!" Mr. Comerford commanded. "Pull over beside the phone box, will you, like a good man." He spoke to her father as if he were his servant.

"Don't you want…?"

"Not yet." Mr. Comerford's voice was firm. "Out you go, Eamon, and take a walk for yourself."

"Eily, come along…"

"No! Just you, Eamon. We'll sit here and chat a little while."

Her father coughed once, twice, hard, and she thought she saw his hand shaking as he pulled up the door handle. She watched as he walked off into the early evening light.

"Now, Eily. Tell me, what would a young good looking girl such as yourself like?"

"I don't know, really."

"Would you fancy a crisp twenty pound note? Think of what you could buy for yourself."

"No thank you." She wanted to get out of the hot back seat.

"No? Well then, how about a nice cool glass of lemonade? I have a fresh bottle here in the picnic basket."

Eily shook her head.

"Well, maybe you'd like to open your blouse for me? You would, wouldn't you?"

Her stomach gurgled. Sweat rose in bubbles on her palms.

"Show me what's under there. Let me drink in your freshness."

Eily leaned towards the window, searching the road for her father, but he was already a ghost faded into the darkening air.

"Come here," Mr. Comerford slowly unbuttoned her cream blouse. He reached under her skirt and drew down her pants, and then her skirt.

"Let me look at you, there's a good girl. Oh…." His voice softened. "Little flowers." He stared at her chest like she was a painting in a museum that he needed to examine down to its finest detail.

"You are immaculate, little girl. Untouched."

How did he know she was pure? She and the angels were the only ones who carried her secret.

"Little flower. Saint Therese of Lisieux, that's you."

For a moment she felt her girl breasts blossoming, petals streaming out of her heart, awash in rainbow shades. She was a flower, and holy too, and finally here was someone who understood. Maybe that's why he was her godfather. Maybe this was God in disguise. But inside, her stomach fought between dread and soft smiles.

"The flower of innocence you are, my child."

He carried his gaze down her body and sighed, "No bird's nest yet, but there will be soon, and that will be that."

He didn't seem bothered by her mottled legs, blotched red and white from hovering over the fire all winter. He was seeing something else entirely.

Eily waited for him to tug at his zipper but he just squirmed in his seat, staring, staring. She thought she saw dampness around his eyes. But when he pulled out a scarlet handkerchief, he only wiped his brow in little, bird like strokes, before passing it to her.

"Here, this is for you, it's from Brown Thomas on Grafton Street, hand woven silk. Now off with you, Eily, go along home. I'll be seeing you soon. Don't forget me."

Eily stumbled out the back door of the car, the handkerchief soaked through. A voice called after her, "And if you see your father, tell him I'm ready for him now."

She went through the front gate, the house looked different to her, smaller somehow. She wasn't ready to go inside. The air had a tinge of muddy green to it, the kind you'd see on a ring that had its silver polished out of it. She crawled into the bushes by the wall and sank onto her hunkers, as she shredded the red, wet square with her teeth.

Mr. Comerford came one more time, several weeks later. Eily heard him and her father exchange heated words in the dining room. As he was leaving, her godfather took her hand in the hallway and looked her up and down, almost sadly. Then he told her she was a big girl now and she never saw or heard from him again. All her father said, when she asked, was there were better ways to make a living than doing business with a man like that.

We're all goin' on a sum-mer holiday. No more working for a week or two. Fun and laugh-ter on our sum-mer holidays. No more worries for me and you. Eily sat in the back of the car, squeezed between Liam and the big suitcase, singing as much of Cliff Richard's song as she could remember. She knew the worries weren't over by a long margin but she let herself be carried along. Maybe the sea would be blue in Port instead of the usual steel gray. Maybe all her dreams would come true one fine day. For now, she hummed until Liam elbowed her in the ribs. "Shurrup, will ye? Me hangover's killing me."

"Liam, you know you shouldn't be drinking like that," her mother clucked but she was laughing. "It'll be the death of you."

Eily continued singing in her head, imagining the angels pitching in though she'd not heard them for a long time now. She was still humming when they pulled into the gravel drive. Lily came scurrying out of the cow shed, a bucket of milk tipped sideways in her hand, a creamy froth flowing over the rim. Dusty the cat raced after it.

"You're early, Eamon." She seemed to be scolding her brother, who just shrugged and parked the car.

"We've a visitor, so we have. D'ye remember Eoghan Butterly from across the way? Well, his first cousin, Johnnie, is over from America. He's inside having a cuppa with Mammy. C'mon in, youse, and meet him."

Eily lashed inside to get a look at the visitor. She'd heard a lot about America in school and she was curious to meet a native.

A round man with a balding head sat next to the fire, his arms resting on the moon of his tummy. "Top o' the mornin' to ye!" He stood up and thrust a hand out but nobody moved to shake it. Eily caught the look of disgust on Liam's face. She felt sorry for the big man and wanted to tell him that nobody talked like that here. Instead she pushed past her father who was blessing himself with holy water from the font by the entryway.

"Glad to meet you..."

"Johnnie they call me, little girl, Johnnie from good ol' Philadelphia!" He spoke loudly as if two voices were coming out of him at once.

"Ah," said her father. "The home of the Liberty Bell."

"That's right, sir. And you must be Eamon, Lily's brother."

Her father nodded slowly.

Fireworks rang in Eily's head when she heard the name, she wasn't sure why. It was as if she'd known those two words forever. "Liberty Bell?" She leaned towards Johnnie. "What's that?"

"Oh, it's a giant bell in Philly," Johnnie sat forward and the rocking chair creaked. "A symbol of freedom, they say."

"Freedom for who?"

"Those who wanted to unshackle themselves from the bondage of England."

Freedom. The word clattered in Eily's chest. She'd not felt such excitement in ages. And isn't that what her own country was after too – separation from the big island? Only they couldn't seem to do it.

"And it has a big crack in it, Eily," her father chipped in.

"It does for sure. Some say we rang it so hard after our victory, we cracked the thing!" Everyone listened as Johnnie let out a roar that might have been laughter.

Eily was enchanted. A country with a bell that rings of freedom, of victory. Lucky the one born in America, she thought.

Silence draped its mantle over the room. Johnnie sat back down and forked up the last of the beans on his plate. Liam coughed long and hard. "You hoovered that up fast enough." He grunted.

Eamon scraped a chair from the table across to the hearth and dropped himself into it. "Ah sure, it's grand to be off my feet. Liam, sit yourself down, why don't you?"

"Well now, if I'm not in the company of a famous rugby hero." Johnnie slugged back his drink. "My mom has all your newspaper clippings. That was a fantastic final win over England at Lansdowne. 14-5…"

"Ah sure, those are long ago days now, aren't they?" Her father was uncomfortable with any talk of his sporting life. "Is there a mug of tea in the house?"

"Coming right up!" Lily had the kettle going in the kitchen. "Young Eily! Would you ever take run over to the Tavern and get us a half pint of ice cream? Neapolitan, I'm thinking. Oh, and some wafers."

"Half pint?" Johnnie looked astonished. "In America, we buy ice cream by the *gallon.*"

Eily felt a ripple of delight seize her body. She couldn't imagine how much a gallon would be. But she loved how everything in America seemed so grand. A place, she imagined, where people were free to express the hugeness of their heart and not squash themselves into tiny cages just so they'd fit in.

America, she tasted the word on her tongue as Lily slipped some change into her hand and she recited it all the way up the High Road to the Tavern. America. America. *Every-body has a summer holiday, doing things they always wanted to....* Some day she'd go there, yes, she surely would.

Out of the sea mist maybe it came but there it was miraging on the path in front of her. The Face. Those nameless eyes that held your entire being in their gaze. Wispy as they were, almost not there, still they lit a fire in Eily's heart that would warm a million winters.

EAMON

The wee county, that's what they called it, where he came from. A stupid name, Eamon thought, even if it was the smallest county in the country. Even Louth riled him, sure, for god's sake, it was too close to lout, given the Irish unwillingness to pronounce their th's. Oh, his wife could do it to perfection, like the Queen of England herself, she sounded. Sometimes it embarrassed him, her velvet accent swanning through the parish when all he wanted was to be quiet, a cipher among the masses. But oh no, off she'd go with her, *I daren't hang out the washing because of the inclement weather* and she always correcting him when he'd say, *I'm just after drying the dishes* or when he'd be wearied to bone and she plaguing him as to what was bothering him, he'd say, *Sure, I'm knackered, amn't I?*

Didn't she know they were expressions carried over from the Irish? Sure, she was useless with the gaeilge. *Fiacla* was the only word she'd try, and that was because it was toothpaste and it was on the top shelf at the chemist's so she had to acknowledge its name.

Well, sure, it was only a metaphor, wasn't it, for the differences between them. Couldn't she understand he wanted to be left alone after a grueling day? It wasn't his fault he found himself in the cool sanctuary of a church when he was going mad driving around the countryside trying to sell insurance policies to a gaggle of blaggards. Who wouldn't want a little comfort here and there when there was hardly a breath of it at home? If it wasn't for the girl, he'd be doomed altogether. And now even she was growing up and off at school most of the time.

A sad old state of affairs, he thought. How had his life turned out like this? The company car would be whisked away from him tomorrow without even an apology. Just like that. As if it was his fault the Irish were so tight with their pennies, they couldn't be bothered investing in calamities that would eventually happen by all accounts.

He wiped the last of the oil off the bicycle chain, sighing. The farming life would have been much closer to his liking. Just him and the teats of cattle. No one to judge or penalize him for what he wasn't even to blame for. Of course, herself'd never have survived in the wee county. The neighbors were always telling him, "Well, isn't your wife a true lady now?" With her high heels and her elegant dresses.

At least she hadn't swollen up like a lot of the women on the road. Heavy with drink and more than their fair share of prataí. She'd kept her figure all right but still he didn't enjoy lying down with her. She didn't have that open way with her body that women should have. Tight as a taut rope, she was, and what could he do to unravel her?

A right mess he'd found himself in. Two children to feed and a cold wife and now, not even the solace of a car he could lock the doors on and be safe for a while. He'd have to get a rain mac if he was to cycle to work, he thought, as he looked at the gloomy sky out the garage door. Sure, what the hell, he might as well have one last jaunt before he had to hand over the keys to his freedom. No point in telling her he was going, she'd only talk him out of it, the forecast being for heavy rains.

He felt almost joyful taking off down the road, like when he was a little boy ambling the country lanes, looking for knockers to bounce off the ground. Sure, he could drive off into forever and leave not a trace if he fancied.

He'd been exhausted, that was the reason. Three days of wheeling around Dublin, door to door begging, that's what it was. "Could I interest you in life insurance, Mrs?" So often recited, he felt like a stuck record. And more often than not, the door shut in his face. This was his last hurrah, he'd drive himself wherever the whim took him. But he'd hardly slept a wink of late and when he caught himself dozing and the car swerved up onto the path on Phibsboro Road, he decided he'd go to the Phoenix Park, find a shady tree to park by and get himself forty winks.

The rains were lashing from the heavens as he drove out past Saint Peter's. He could hardly see through the wipers, the windows all fogged up and the rain pelting against the glass.

Get me there in one piece, God, he sang to himself, as he inched down the road, giving the lorry ahead of him a good breadth. *I'll make everything up to you, I swear I will.* He was relieved when he saw the park's monument on his right. He was close now. The first decent spot he found, he'd take it.

And there it was: a huge oak with branches dripping over the footpath. Shelter. He pulled in under it, turned off the ignition, and in a few minutes, he was settling into himself. Cosy it felt with the water pinging off the car roof. He could stay here forever.

Then it happened: one minute, he was leaning back against the car seat, eyes closed, his breathing slowing, and the next, a godforsaken clatter and the car kangarooing up in the air and crashing back down again. Glass in smithereens daggering into his clenched hands.

"Holy Mother of God!" His breath on fire. Half of the oak tree had crashed onto the front of the car, the windshield in tatters, and his skin tingling with embedded shards of glass.

One more inch, everyone had said, and you'd have been a goner. Someone was looking after you. Not the gods of money, anyway. At least the car was insured, being in the business he was. But old Casey the manager'd be down his throat about it, as if he was to blame. In a way, he wished he'd parked a couple of feet closer to the tree but when he imagined it, everything became blurry and he could see only gray mud.

EILY

Her father was fuming so hard, spit was firing out of his mouth when Eily walked in. "That black bastard!" He shook what looked like a letter out into the air as if it contained the answer to everything, and it wasn't the right answer. "He *promised* me! He promised me!" On he raged.

"What's the matter, Daddy?" Eily reached her arms out to him. Her father continued pacing and muttering, half curses snaking out from his lips.

"Daddy?"

Eventually, he flung the letter on the kitchen table.

"Eily, my uncle Jack died in hospital last week. In his sleep, if you don't mind."

"Oh Daddy, I'm sorry for your loss." She knew it was what people said at times like this: *condolences,* they called it. And besides, it hurt her heart to see her father so upset.

"You needn't bother with that," he said. "Good riddance to him, the blaggard! The old man said he'd leave me his boxing money, his estate, the lot. A colossal sum it was."

"I remember…"

"Well, he's gone and changed his mind at the last minute – or someone changed it for him! The whole stash is going to Lily now. And we without even a car to our name."

Aunt Lily still lived in the big stone house in Port. Eily knew that Lily grew vegetables and flowers and sold them at the Saturday market in Dunleer, but her father said she didn't need the money, only to occupy her time.

"I just do *not* believe it!" Her father was circling round the kitchen. "After what he did…" His voice trailed off as he leveled his black boot at the door, chipping yellow paint and dinging the wood.

"Wait till your mother gets home!" His voice like a threat. "Here, give me that letter." Though Eily hadn't touched it.

He tore at the thick paper, shredding it into pieces, swung open the back door, and flung the white bits out on the air. "Let the birds have it!"

Eily sat in the laundry room till after midnight, as he and her mother whispered in the kitchen. "Eamon, I'll take a bus to Drogheda and ask you-know-who for a loan. That could get us through…"

They argued back and forth about it, but next day, her mother got up early, had her boiled egg and marmalade toast eaten, dishes washed, by the time Eily came downstairs.

She had her best suit on, a green tweed she brought over from England after she married. Her hair was done up in a neat bun.

"How do I look?" She didn't do her usual full turn, only patted powder on her cheeks in the mirror. Though she was always elegant, Eily thought she looked a bit severe. "Lovely, Mum," she offered.

Her mother picked up her red handbag, tucked a cloth hanky inside, and as she walked out the door, she said, "You can warm the fish fingers for supper, Eily. I need to go away for a day or two."

Eily nodded, wondering if she was off to see Miss Coughlan, who'd come into a tidy sum, she knew, after she'd gone to America and worked as a housekeeper for a rich man for twenty years. When he died, he'd left her his house and belongings. She had sold them and come back to Ireland and had the stone house built for Eily's father's family so they could move out of the cottage on the high road. That was where her Uncle Nick had fallen out the half door and maybe gotten the T.B. that killed him.

Eily soon found out she was right when her mother came home a day later, her eyes rimmed with red.

"Go outside, Eily, and play now." Her father nudged her onto the back step, but she held her ear to the door.

"She wouldn't do it, would she?"

Silence.

"Eamon, all she said was, 'why did he have to go and marry a Sasanach anyway?'"

Eily was rummaging through the writing desk for a pencil when she came across the vellum stationery she'd bought for her mother that wild, rainy day in Eason's. She opened it carefully, wanting to run her fingers along the lavender paper, it was so pretty. On top, she saw a letter in her mother's handwriting. She found it hard to read, the letters were so small, but with effort, she could decipher it like a code.

To the attention of William Casey, General Manager
Norwich Union Insurance
Dawson Street
Dublin 2

Dear Mr. Mackey,
I appreciate that my husband Eamon Massey was not promoted to Head of Sales, although he was highly qualified. I am sure you had a number of worthy candidates. He has had some challenges with sales on the road, I concede, but they did not interfere with his capacity to fulfill his duties. He has met his quota and even exceeded it for the past two years. It is my express wish and request that, regardless of my husband's religious excesses, you keep him on at the Norwich.
We have two children and a third on the way and are completely dependent on his income. I hope you will find it in your heart to appreciate our situation. My husband values his career with you and I can assure you he is a dedicated worker.
Thank you for your kind consideration.

Eily read and re-read the letter, the words spinning round in her head. She sat down next to the telephone, her hands shaking. If she asked her mother, she'd know she'd been reading something she shouldn't and yet she was desperate for answers.

Finally, she opted for honesty, a rare thing in that household. "Mum," she entered the kitchen quietly where her mother was putting egg yolk on the Cornish pasties. "Mum... are we going to have another baby?"

Her mother raised an eyebrow. "How did you know? Did Daddy tell you?"

"No, I... I came across your letter."

Her mother plucked it quickly out of Eily's hand, yellow liquid seeping into the paper. "How on earth...! Well, it doesn't matter now. The secret is out. Yes, Eily," she sighed. "You'll be having a little brother or sister soon."

Eily flung her arms around her mother. "Oh Ma, brilliant!"

Her mother touched Eily's hair for a second, then brushed her away. "We shall see."

Eily twirled around the room, arms out, almost knocking down the milk jug on the sideboard. "If you want to move like that, go out into the garden and celebrate with Mrs. Mulligan."

Her mother had told her years ago that an old woman called Mrs. Mulligan lived in the lilac bush and often sent her out there to have a chat. "Will she talk to me, d'ye think?" Eily had asked, for most old people she knew kept their heads down and bodies held tight and would never look at you.

"Oh, you're a dreamer. I'm sure she'll respond."

Eily had spent many a happy hour out on the upturned laundry bucket, chatting a mile a minute to Mrs. M., who hadn't much to say but was a really good listener. Now that she had turned eleven, Eily knew that she was talking to the flowers really. But it felt soothing to have someone to share herself with.

"I will go, Ma, and tell her about the baby. But first, I have to ask, why are you asking for Daddy to have his job kept?"

"Don't call me Ma."

"Sorry."

"It's nothing to worry about, Eileen. We just want to be sure we can keep a roof over our heads for the next decade." Her mother put the pasties in the oven. "Besides, I won't be posting that letter now. It's completely stained. I'll have to go in person." She moved

Eily towards the back door. "Tell Mrs. Mulligan the good news, why don't you?"

"C'mere till I tell you," a short girl with an elastic face ran after Eily as she was leaving the classroom. "You live up on Glasilawn by the phone box, don't you?"

Eily nodded in surprise. She wasn't used to anyone at school talking to her.

"Well, I live on The Extension. That's just round the block from you, isn't it?"

Eily nodded again. The girl started keeping step with her and they walked up through Cremore together. "You see that house?"

Eily looked over at the gray stone house across the road. "C'mere. Stand beside me. Now, what do you see at the top of the stairs?"

Eily looked through the glass window above the front door. There was something tall and white on the landing.

"It's a statue." The girl said. "But some say that it moves because the house is haunted."

Eily felt a thrill slide through her. The house did look a little worse for wear, as her mother would say. Weeds were peeking out through the iron fence and onto the footpath.

"Have you seen it move?"

"Oh yeah, many's the time. If we wait long enough, it'll happen. Sit down beside me, why don't you?"

Eily sat on the low wall as the girl pulled out a packet of Wrigley's from her schoolbag. "Here, have a stick." It was spearmint and it tingled Eily's tongue.

"You know me, don't ye?"

"Yeah, you're Kiara Moran. I saw you win the sprint last year at the races."

Kiara laughed. "Yeah, I pretend I've got a cop chasing me and that gets me going!"

"Well, he must have been an angry cop cos you were really fast."

"G'way outta that."

Eily could tell she was pleased. Kiara had the look of an athlete. Her face and body were loose as she moved. She cracked each of her fingers in turn and then her thumbs.

"Well, I saw you topple over when you tried to stand on your hands."

It was Eily's turn to laugh. "I tried but the ground just wouldn't hold me."

"You're gas," Kiara spat out her gum. "Hey lookit! Did ye see that?"

Eily looked up quickly at the statue but it was still as stone.

"Ah well, next time. You want to walk home again tomorrow?"

"Brilliant!"

"Okay, I'll see you at three outside the gate."

Every day after that, Eily met her new friend after school and they'd saunter home, stopping to sit on a wall here and there to rest. Kiara insisted on walking Eily to her house and then Eily would return the favor. They'd walk each other home back and forth until the sky draped its dark cloak over the neighborhood.

Kiara got pocket money every Friday. Eily knew better than to ask for it at home and was surprised when Kiara took her into Whitty's one afternoon and bought each of them an Ice Burger. She almost fell over herself hugging Kiara.

"Get off me, you!" Kiara pushed her away. "It's only an ice cream. When I buy you a Cortina, then you can hug me!" And they laughed, licking the melting cream between two biscuits.

Sister Avril, the new, pink-faced nun, rapped the desk with her ruler. Each thwack echoed through the room, pinging off the loose windows. "I have an announcement, young ladies." She was young and pretty and though her voice was raised, she had the look of a fragile deer. Air seemed to whistle through her mouth as she spoke. "I'm offering a special prize for the girl who writes the best essay on 'My Summer Holidays.'"

Eily still adored writing. She'd read her way through most of Drumcondra library and loved how magic happened so easily in books. It was the one place you could feel powerful, where you could sit down with a pencil and make anything happen. But summer holidays – what could she say about that? Long days with more light and maybe the odd gift of sunshine but the family hardly ever went anywhere except Port.

"It's due on Thursday morning, girls, so get writing."

Eily spent the afternoon straining for a story that would light up the page. On the way out of geography class, she heard Mairead Flynn talking about how her parents had taken her to the Continent in July for a fortnight. It was hot, she heard Mairead say, and how she'd gotten sunburned on her nose and everyone spoke in a foreign language. Eily had no idea where the Continent was, or even what it was. But a spark ignited inside her and she hardly heard Kiara chatting away as they walked home.

As soon as she got in the door, she made a beeline for the dining room table and out poured her make believe holiday. She took along with her her new best friend and her dreamed-up family as they soared through the air to a place where all wishes came true.

Eily was smiling by the time she ran out of words. It was almost as good as really going. She decided it was time to write something longer, where you didn't have to stop, but let the letters unfurl like angel wings on the snowy page that could fly on forever. A novel, she thought, her eyes gleaming.

They weren't even finished with homework when Mr. Moran pushed open the door.

"Time to go, Kiara."

"Where?" Eily was surprised.

"Oh, our da is taking us to Portrane strand. It's Wally's birthday and we're taking a picnic out there."

"Ah," Eily picked up her pencil and jotter. "Well, I'll be off then."

"Sure, wait, why don't you, till we're all in the car." Kiara loved to talk and Eily was all ears.

"I will then."

Eily stood on the road and watched as all seven children packed themselves into the orange Volkswagen Beetle *2609 Z*. Eily memorized license plates for enjoyment. It was a lovely car, unusual in these parts, like a magic bubble. She could hardly believe so many bodies could fit inside it. Mr. Moran at the wheel and his wife next to him, the toddler twins on her lap. She thought of them all lounging in the sand, sandcastles and moats at their feet.

"Happy Birthday, Wally!" She shouted and waved after the car as it took off down the road, though she was close to tears. She'd only been to the sea once, back when she was seven and her mother had been fed up about something. She'd said, "Blow it!" and rung for a taxi and shoveled Liam and herself into the back seat. The wind was whipping sand up on their bare legs and into their sandwiches. She remembered swinging in a little blue boat, goose pimpled but grateful to watch the gray water dance. She just kept waving, trying to smile.

She was closing the garden gate when she saw it: the little orange car doing a quick turnaround at the end of the street. And it was heading directly towards her.

Eily wondered what they'd forgotten.

"You!" Mr. Moran rolled down his window. "Get in, would ye? We couldn't leave you behind and you looking so downcast. Besides, we're into autumn now. How many warm days have we left?"

"But..." Eily couldn't see how she could possibly squeeze in to the packed car.

"The shelf, girl, the back shelf," Mr. Moran got out and opened the boot. "Tuck yourself up in there, why don't you?"

Eily crawled into the tiny space above the back seat, grinning through the rear window like a Cheshire cat.

Visions of golden sand sifting through her toes and the icy tingle of sea water on her skin had Eily in a trance. The girls were already seated at their desks but Eily's head was brimming with the beauty of that endless liquid that took her in and held her. She drifted slowly towards her chair.

"Eileen Massey! Come here to me now!" Sister Avril's whistling voice wrenched Eily out of her beautiful dream. Her heart chugged in her chest. What kind of trouble was she in now?

Her limbs shaky as she moved through the aisle up to the desk.

Sister Avril stood up and Eily almost offered her hand for a rap. But no, the nun pulled out a jotter, flicking through the pages until she came to what she was after.

"This here, girls," she sounded like the breeze in the trees, "is what an essay should be. 'My Summer Holidays' was a joy to read, surprising, funny, and it kept me on my toes. Who wouldn't want a holiday where wishes drip off trees and the weather is always perfect? Eily," she opened her desk drawer. "You're the winner of my contest. Here you go."

Eily held her hand out and a large box of Cadbury's Milk Tray chocolates landed in it. She was breathless, adjusting slowly to being praised instead of punished. Especially as nuns were supposed to want nothing from this world but their husband, God.

She took the chocolates and a few girls clapped.

Kiara was delighted with the bounty. "Les-see..." and she peeled off the plastic wrapper, hastily prying open the box. "Jesus Mary and Josephine, there's two layers in there!"

Eily told her to help herself, glad to be able to share something with her friend who'd been so generous. "Take as many as you want."

Eily watched as Kiara plucked out one, then another, biting delicately on the chocolate coating and letting the cherry or almond filling drip onto her tongue. "Let's have a sit down now on the wall here and enjoy them."

"You were always one for the words, weren't ye?"

"Suppose so."

"Well, I'm always one for the sweets!"

They spent the afternoon sauntering homewards, taking a break at a wall here and there, another chocolate at each stop. By the time they got to Ballygall Road, three sweets remained. "Listen, we can have one more each," Eily handed her friend the coconut swirl. "But I better keep one just to prove to my ma that I won."

Kiara nodded, her lips rimmed in brown. "God, she'll be so proud of you. Brains run in your tribe, don't they? I mean, Liam and all."

Eily shrugged and folded the lid down. Liam was already getting tutoring for university but Eily didn't think herself brainy at all. More heart-y, she thought. When she got home, it was almost dark and her mother looked at the almost empty box. "You won't want your supper now, will you?" And she pointed to the dustbin. "Put the remains in there when you're finished."

Old Maher from Drogheda delivered kerosene once a month. Hefting the blue tank off his lorry, he'd wheeze a bit, have to catch his breath and Eily would stand close by to help as he struggled to lug his wares towards the garage. Eily wondered how such a slight man would undertake such a heavy job. On his way out, he'd always raise his cap and tell her what a fine young woman she was becoming.

Eily doubted that. She couldn't concentrate in school. The year's end exams were coming up and she hadn't studied a tap. It was her mother's fault, always telling her to be quiet because Liam was studying. "You don't tell him to be quiet for me," Eily had said.

"That's because you're a girl, Eily, and you'll get married one day. You won't need an education then. And another thing. When you do marry, please, dear, just elope."

Eily vowed to herself she'd never get married. Boys were more a nuisance than anything. Her father was already taken and Liam still treated her like a child.

She found herself spilling out her sad story to old Maher, who leaned against the hedge, his head tipped to one side so his cap almost slid off. "I'm sorry for your trouble, Eily. Your mam only wants the best for you, I'd wager. It's hard enough these days to raise a daughter."

"Thanks, Mr. Maher," Eily was grateful for the way he listened, carefully, as if every word she shared was important.

"Ah, call me Jamesie, would you? Isn't that my name after all? You're making me feel like an old codger."

And they both laughed for he must have been seventy at least. Eily thought she could hear a rattling in his chest and she worried what troubles he must have of his own.

"Have you a family yourself, Mr. Maher?"

"Not a one," he sighed, then brightened, "and maybe I'm better off for that!"

"You might be right! If I lived alone, I'd never worry about bills and arguments, only write stories all day long."

Whatever it was in Maher's easy manner, Eily couldn't help but pour out her heart to him. She told him about the prize she'd won for her essay on the summer holidays and how now she was thinking about writing an actual novel.

Maher raised an eyebrow in surprise. "Well, well, isn't that a marvelous thing. And at your age. Maybe sometime – when you're ready, of course – you'd read me a bit of it. In the old days, I was fond of the books."

"Maybe sometime I will." Eily felt more cheerful that she had in a long time. Someone interested in her just because. She waved Maher off into the afternoon with a wide smile.

Eily was disappointed when Liam ditched the newsagent's to sign on with the FCA. He said, better a volunteer army than none at all. He was away most weekends, leaving only Mrs. Mulligan for her to talk to and now that she was almost a teenager, it wasn't so thrilling anymore. Liam'd take off on his Honda 50 in his fatigues and spend two nights at the barracks. He told everyone at supper that he could shoot a bullseye with the rifle they gave him every time.

When he was home, he spent most of the day on his bed, reading about Home Rule and eating Corn Flakes out of the box with his hands. He hardly looked at Eily, and then only to toss out a curse word he was fond of or a slag to try and rile her. Come dusk, he'd be leaning against the garage wall with his gaggle of friends, cigarettes braced in the hinge of their mouths, and they'd slap each other on the back, cackling and spitting wads of phlegm across the garden. Through the washroom curtain, Eily would watch the smoke swirling round them, clouds of dim light floating up on the gray air.

She wished they could see the iron clamps wedged in their chests, that she could unhook them and let in the soft light that was her intimate. She sighed as they slouched before her in their army fatigues, all guff and banter, sad for the hardnesses they clutched tight to themselves.

And now her mother was ripe with child again; her stomach swelled like Jackie Charlton's football. She hardly spoke of it, only slowed sometimes to catch her breath. One evening, Eily found her on the sitting room couch, peeling a mandarin. The thin blue curtains were drawn, and the fire weak in the hearth. The television was blaring News at Ten like it always did. Her mother watched television while they were praying, and always turned the sound down if her father walked in, especially when there were ads for women's under garments.

Eily sat at her mother's feet, close to the warmth of the hearth.

"Would you like a wedge, Eily?"

"No thanks, but I'd love to feed one to the baby."

Eily couldn't believe her mother would allow her to peel crescents off the orange and slide it into her mother's mouth. "One for love." she would say. "Two for health. Three for the angels."

"That's enough, Eily. The baby is still small, it needs oxygen more than food."

But Eily, charmed as she was to be as close to her mother, knew it was talk of angels that brought the sweet moment to a swift end. Her mother had no interest in fantasy, as she called it. She was too busy cooking, cleaning, sewing, shopping. Who had time for angels these days?

Sometimes Eily's heart hurt when she watched Kiara's mother sing while she made supper. *Will you still feed me, will you still need me when I'm 64?* She'd toss her head back, laughing. And all eight of the Morans would squeeze around the long table in the kitchen, everyone talking at once, not a bother on any of them.

Mrs. Moran had even read Eily's essay about her holiday on the Continent and had sat her down in their living room one afternoon. "You've got the makings of a writer, girl," she peered over her black rimmed glasses.

"Thanks a million," Eily could feel her face pinkening. "I'd love to be Enid Blyton The Second, actually. I've read nearly all her books."

"No," Mrs. Moran had been firm. "You would not. Why not be Eileen Massey The First?"

Eily loved that idea. Not being in anyone's shadow, even her idol. She beamed all the way home. She couldn't even stop to eat, only sit herself down on the sagging couch, pencil in hand, and start writing her first novel. It would be about a girl, Nessa, she decided, with a river of auburn hair flowing down her back just like her name sounded. She'd have a spell put on her so she was helpless but to always speak the truth. Eily would have a field day dreaming up all the trouble that would cause. Her first sentence leaped onto the page. *Nessa knew what priests really do, there would be no more secrets.*

She was smiling to herself all evening long, hardly noticing that her mother wasn't in the kitchen cooking, that no one had called her to tea. When Eily looked up from her jotter, she realized how quiet the house was. Not even a breeze outside ruffling the hedges. Everyone was probably at Mass, it was Holy Thursday after all. Maybe that was what Jesus meant by the Last Supper, she sighed, and went back to her writing. She hoped old Maher would come around again soon. She could trust him, she knew, with the truth.

Good Friday, they called it. The day to fast and offer up all your sins to God. Eily came running down the stairs, taking them two at a time, and almost fell over her mother as she turned into the hallway.

"Eily! Out of the way," her father pushed her into the kitchen. "The ambulance'll be here any minute." He kept a firm grip on the door handle and all Eily could do was listen to the siren screaming out on the street, the loud knock on the door, a mad shuffling in the hallway.

"Lord have mercy." A man's voice. "Good thing you rang soon as you did."

"She just keeled over," her father's voice, faltering, and then the door handle loosening. "Said her woman parts hurt."

Eily ran out just in time to see her mother on a stretcher being hefted into the back of the ambulance. "Mummy! Mummy!

What's wrong?" Her eyes were closed and she seemed to be barely breathing.

"Stop it, Eily. Leave her be."

She stood watching her mother disappearing from her, turning at the end of the road by the post box, the siren quieting, and then gone.

She slouched back through the garden gate and into the house, tears of blood streaked across the carpet. Eily fell onto her knees, trying to lick up every last drop.

For days, her mother's name was not mentioned. Although the shoes were still polished and the prayers said at night, there was no porridge warming on the stove in the mornings, no soup when she came in for dinner. Eily took to opening each drawer of her mother's dressing table and inhaling her lavender sachets and soaps from England. Each whiff reminded Eily of what was missing. She knew she wouldn't trade her mother for Mrs. Moran, no matter how jolly she was. *Come home, Ma, please,* she whispered on the evening air.

Once the nuns found out her mother was in hospital, they brought her over to their living quarters and forced hot cocoa down her throat. Eily hated the thick scum of scalded milk on the top, and retched when she tried to swallow. But they made her drink every last drop.

Some evenings, when her father came in from selling insurance policies, he'd stick a steak and kidney pie in the oven and tell Eily to keep an eye on it. Once he tried making peelers, re-fried potatoes he said his own mother used to make. Every slice of bread he toasted came out charred, but he'd only laugh and say the black bits were good for your teeth.

His nightly visits became shorter, more abrupt, no lullaby, just a firm hand guiding hers to the place of no return. She still came down afterwards to the garden but when she tried to dance, her hips felt stiff, her legs heavy. No sign of the moon, only a glut of gray clouds leering from overhead.

Kiara had her eye on one of the lads but she wouldn't say who. She'd pretend not to notice when they were holding up the wall down by the Tolka. One of them would shout, "Howaya, young one!" and Kiara would raise a brow and laugh. Eily couldn't understand why boys were so important when her mother was sick in hospital.

One Saturday, the gang was huddled against the rain on the corner of Mobhi road, some rough looking types alongside. They'd found a pool of tadpoles and had been catching them and slicing them with a penknife.

"I'd lay a tenner on youse being too scaredy-cat to even touch them!" A short boy with missing teeth jeered.

"Little Leeper!" Kiara shouted at him. "We'll show you."

And she marched Eily home to get their wellies and a bucket. "C'mon, it'll be brilliant," she said.

But once they got to the pool, they saw hundreds of tadpoles spooling around in a mess of dark water and muck. Eily imagined her mother, the puddles of blood oozing round her.

"Yuck, they're so slimy." Kiara pinched her nose, though it wasn't the tadpoles that smelled so much as the litter decaying in the river.

Eily cheered up, seeing the creatures swimming so smoothly when they were all packed together in a tiny hole. "How could they knife them, Kiara, poor little things. I know! Let's catch one and bring it home in a bucket and wait for it to turn into a frog."

"Yeah," Kiara was sulking. "And then we can kiss him and he'll become a bleedin' prince."

"Oh c'mon…" But as soon as Eily caught one, it slipped out of her fingers and back into its murky home. She got down on her knees in the mud and plucked a long gray one out. It was too fast for her. Eily dived into the water after it, making a big splash, her hands feathered in mud. She wiped her face and loose strands of her hair became thick and heavy.

"It's no use, Kiara," Eily laughed. "Well, maybe it's for the best. Leave them where they belong."

"Looks like you belong in there too," Kiara said, hauling the empty bucket up the hill. The rain plastered Eily's hair to her face. She felt alive for the first time in ages, a thrill riddling her body. "That was a laugh."

"You're got a strange sense of humor, then." Kiara was in no mood to joke around.

The lads were waiting at the top of Cremore Drive. "Did yis find any?" Declan Arnold asked. He was the gentle one of the pack but he looked downtrodden, like a dog who'd been left out in the cold too long. Eily felt sorry for him.

"Would you look at the state of ye!" someone said to Eily. "Tadpoles try to drown you, did they?"

"Ladies, I've a tadpole of me own you can have any time," Little Leeper pushed his torso forward.

The boys cackled and Eily watched sadly as Kiara combed her hair with her fingers. "Do I look all right?" She whispered. Eily nodded and the happiness leaked out the back door of her heart in one flush. Her best friend was choosing boys over her.

When she slouched in the back door, her father took one look and sent her upstairs to take a bath. "As your mother would say, if she were here, God help her, you look like the wreck of the Hesperus."

The stairs creaked under her soggy shoes. The house was hollow without her.

Eily swished the luke warm water in the tub, pouring a pan of it over her head, sighing. She missed her mother's cooking, the sound of oil spitting in the frying pan, bread warming in the oven. Sundays was always Toad-In-The-Hole. Gooey Yorkshire pud with tiny cocktail sausages sunken into it and a smear of Gye over the top. But tonight, all she could think of were those tadpoles waiting to flower into frogs, not sausages swimming in batter and her appetite was only for sleep.

She woke in the night, though, her heart pounding, and sat up in bed. Was it a bad dream? Her father was snoring in the back room. She turned on the light and reached for her pencil and jotter. She'd let Nessa talk to her, calm her down. Nessa never lied. Chapter 2, she wrote. *What fathers do when they are lonely or sad.*

She was still writing, her left hand cramping up, when she heard Liam slamming the back door. He must have a day off from the barracks, she thought, opening the curtain to welcome the brightening sky.

Her father was already in the sitting room, blowing into the weak fire, when she came down. He didn't turn around. "I've a few policies to sort out in Wicklow. Lord knows why people can't read the fine print. Don't wait up for me, all right?"

For a second, Eily felt a twinge, her father leaving too, but it was faint. The room of her heart was filling up with Nessa and her fierce honesty. If her new companion didn't compromise or cave in, why should she?

She put the kettle on. "Want a cuppa, Liam?"

He grunted, head bent over the newspaper. "Mm."

She put the pot on the table, milk and sugar next to it. "It's steeping. Help yourself when you're ready." She slathered butter on the last of her mother's bread.

"Have to go," Liam shoved his chair back. His friends were coming round by the coal house. It was always the same. The lot of them would troop into the garage. Only last week, someone had brought a can of paint. Another hefted a ladder inside. She'd leaned against the closed door, trying to hear what they were saying, but all she heard was a mess of curses and hacking laughter.

They almost knocked her over when the door opened finally. "Would you look at that? She wants to join the gang, lads!'

"I do not!"

"Send her off to the Army first, for a bit of training."

"Well, what are you eavesdropping on us for then, girl?"

"Get in the house! Now!" Liam's hand on her arm, dragging her into the kitchen, and she lurching after him, yelling.

Eily went back upstairs and launched Nessa into her third chapter. *What boys really want and what girls think they do.* She didn't feel lonely when Nessa was nattering on in her knowing way. It was like having a companion who could talk your ear off, only you wanted her to. Both ears, even.

As evening opened it arms, Liam brought his friends inside to the sitting room and came back to Eily in the kitchen. "Didn't I tell you to make yourself scarce when me mates are here?"

"But where'd I go?"

"I don't want you around them. There'll only be trouble."

"But I'll be quiet. I'll go upstairs."

"No. It's under the stairs for you, Ugly, or outside."

"It's cold out there. I'll be good, so I will."

"Then it's under the stairs," he opened the hatch door. The hairs on Eily's wrists grew taut.

"No, not there, please...."

"I don't have time for this messing. It's for your own good." And out he shoved Eily into the darkening garden as the boys trooped in.

The back door, yellow paint peeling, her small fingers clawing. Somewhere a voice screaming, was it an *aisling* come floating through the ethers, a voice scratching the heavens, it seemed so far away, *Let me in! Let me in! Let me...*

Rains howling down, gutter overspilling, hair glutted on cheek, and all lines to heaven down. Table, chairs, stool wedged against the inside of the door, as if she could possibly break through.

The taunting jeers through that vital slab of wood – the bridge between belonging and despair – didn't hurt as much as the chill. Skin goosebumped, white, blue, and her throat raw as a sliced finger. Thumbs bloodied as she sank to her knees, keeling back onto the concrete.

She crawled to the garage door, and hunkered next to the

drainpipe. She'd be out for the night now. No mother to cry No. Father away on his insurance rounds.

Eily thought she saw a whisper of moon through the brute sky as she skimmed, a slug, on her knees across the grass, and settled under the apple tree, her true mother, and slept.

The back door was ajar when Eily woke up. She'd heard the thrum of Liam's motorbike revving up but had dozed through it. He was gone. Eily hooshed herself up to sitting, shivering. It had rained in the night and her cardigan was sagging like a damp sponge. She faltered inside and upstairs and ran a bath. The drenched dress was a sort of comfort to her, even as she took it off. She'd felt that way when she'd come home from the fields last year, her cheek slit from a broken bottle and found Grandma from England waiting for her in the hallway. She was made to take every stitch off because she was soaked through. She'd resisted Grandma's firm hand, wanting the cool consolation of her clothes.

"Mark my words, Eily, you'll get arthritis if you stay in that outfit. I've seen it happen." Grandma had scolded her but in a gentle way. She was a delicate lady who made women's hats and always wore a tailored dress. Eily was supposed to take after her, with her blue eyes and easy face. Eily wondered how she could know so much when her daughter was always taking the ferry to England to look after her.

When her mother had asked about the gash on her cheek, Eily said she'd fallen on a broken milk bottle. But even now, she knew that wasn't true. No one pushed her for another answer and she filed it away in the back pocket of her mind until she couldn't even remember herself.

She lay down in the warm bath, letting her hair trail out behind her. She adored water, how it always made room for you, no matter your size, how it had no edges and didn't object to your presence, only folded you into it arms like a kind mother.

She heard the kitchen door slam below and sat up. Her father was shouting up the stairs at her. She grabbed a towel and wrapped it around her.

"Come down here now, Eily. I have news."

Eily pulled on her white vest and pants and went down to the kitchen. Her father and Liam were sitting at the table. Liam looked scared. Her father had his head in his hands.

"Liam and Eily, your mother lost the babby. We didn't want to say anything until we knew for certain." Her father's voice kept breaking like a bad telephone line. "It was a boy. We named him Robert Joseph on account… on account of his due date falling on St. Joseph's Day."

"He was alive…?" Eily's eyes widened.

"He was, but only for a few hours. Poor lad came out too early and he'd a hard time getting enough oxygen."

Eily's eyes welled up in tears. "Oh, little creature… How's Mum?"

"Very tired, Eily. She's in convalescent care at the minute and we don't know how long she'll be there. They're going to…" her father's voice broke into a hundred pieces, "to… to remove her mothering parts."

"What do you mean, Daddy?"

"She had cancer, didn't she?" Liam said, serious for once. He wanted to be an army medic and he knew things you wouldn't expect from a teenager. He was already taking university classes with a tutor in Ballsbridge.

"Yes, of the womb. We'll not be having any more babies now." He looked like he'd been crushed by a ten-foot lorry.

"I knew it!" Liam banged his fist on the table.

"God is punishing us."

"Oh Daddy," Eily couldn't help but put her arms around her father's quaking shoulders. "It's not a punishment. Mum is alive and she'll get better, won't she?"

Her father half nodded. "Eily, pull down the beads, will you? We'll all kneel down now and say the Rosary together."

Afterwards, Eily's father rummaged in his pocket and pulled out a fiver. "Liam, go up to Casoni's and get us all a cod and chips. Sure, there'll be no cooking in this house tonight."

Liam seemed glad to leave what had the air of a funeral and he took off on his Honda 50.

After they'd peeled away the wax paper and eaten in silence, Eily's father said he'd be away for a few days. "Business up in Louth. Liam, you take care of the girl, will you?"

Liam mumbled under his breath.

"I can take care of myself! I'm old enough now and can do a better job than some people..."

Her father packed some shirts and ties in the old brown suitcase and he was out the door.

Liam and Eily stared at each other for a minute. Then Liam took the stairs in twos, locked his bedroom, and put a record on. *You can leave here for four days in space but when you return it's the same old place...* Eily knew the song well. It was her brother's favorite. She listened to Eve of Destruction from downstairs over and over and over until she fell asleep at the table.

EAMON

He was no more going to Louth than the man in the moon. It was the last place he wanted to be. Strange how that's what slipped out. Like the feckin' salmon, you always ended up back where you began. But it wasn't home to him, never was. Dublin wasn't much better. Trapped, that's how he felt. What if he lost her, if she was too far gone to rally round? He didn't have it in him to raise Eily. Liam'd be out of the house soon enough. But there'd always be a hole there, the boy they should have had, the one that would have brought them together.

God must be rejoicing now, he thought, getting back at him for his sins. Not loving the wife enough, complaining about his job, lashing out at Liam for his sullen cheek. And the girl. What could he do, couldn't help himself, she was the only one cared a halfpenny bit for him, an ounce of comfort for all his pain. She never asked him to stop, did she? Heaven knows, he loved her, a slice of sunshine in the grim rounds of disappointment, how she welcomed him in from the cold, listened to his stories. She was a grand girl, his *chailín álainn*. Who could begrudge him that?

Maybe it was penace for herself taking the Pill all those years but he hadn't known, had he? No one could blame him for that. And for God's sake, he wasn't making excuses, but look what Uncle Jack'd done. Ruined him forever. Not a moment's peace since that day in the field. And after all that, he'd bloody well gone and betrayed him in the end. Hadn't he prayed and wept and prayed till his throat hurt, lost the company car only because he was always stopping off in churches to light a candle and offer up his sins? Was this his penance, the Lord's way of tormenting him? He'd do anything to make up, anything. He'd find a way to get back into His graces, so he would. He'd think of something.

But now everything was falling apart. He was barely holding down the day job. His head was a muddle as he climbed onto the 34. The bus was almost full but he snagged a seat next to an old woman, her lap full of groceries. When she finally got off, he leaned in close to the window and let the passing houses and shops disappear.

At the terminus, he gave a nod to the driver, said he was staying on. All day he rode into town and back out again until the gray of sky muted to black. He couldn't go home yet, couldn't face the pair of them, or himself. He pulled the few bills and spare change out of his trouser pocket, counted it, and bartered a room for himself above the Gravediggers pub. A thin sheet stretched over him, up to his chin, a mummy, and he was out for the count.

EILY

Two days passed and no sign of their father. Liam mostly ignored Eily and stayed put in his room.

Someone in school said that May Day was the first day of spring; Eily usually liked having a birthday when the whole world was beginning to blush into bloom. Even the crew cut grass in the back garden seemed to reach taller. When she was younger, she would circle the driveway on her tricycle, waiting for the postman, dreaming of all the treats he might be carrying in his haversack for her. Over the years, she had gotten used to the lone card from Grandma in England, the sixpence from her mother and the bewilderment of her father when he discovered it was his daughter's special day. And today, everyone had forgotten her age had just turned the dial past twelve. She was a teenager now. Who cared about the sixpence? She'd trade it for her mother coming home any day of the year.

Maybe after breakfast, she'd scour the garden for a crocus or even an apple leaf, something to mark the day, even if no one else noticed or cared. Or she'd have Nessa write a chapter just for her, *Birthday Treats for All-Alone Girls.*

She was helping herself to a jam sandwich when she heard the grinding sound of a tired engine turning over. It was stopped outside the house by the phone box. She ran to the gate and found Maher sitting at the wheel, chewing on his tobacco.

"Maher... I mean Jamesie!" she shouted through the window. "You're back again."

Maher waved and slowly eased himself out of the driver's seat. "Tis no lie, Eily. Only I've to keep the engine running so it doesn't conk out altogether. The lorry's getting on, just like myself."

Eily pressed her palms over her ears, smiling. "Leave it be, then, and come on in."

Maher followed her into the sitting room. "Have you need of kerosene, today?" He asked, coughing into a soiled hankie.

"I don't think so. Sure, we're into May now. It's only me and my brother here anyway and we wear extra jumpers when it's cold. But as you're here, why don't you warm yourself by the hearth?" Eily said it as a way of comforting the man who looked ill even though the fire had not been lit. "Can I get you a cuppa?"

Maher rubbed his hands together, nodding. "Sounds ideal, love."

Eily felt almost grown up as she carried in the tin tray from England, two steaming mugs of Lyons tea and a Welsh Rarebit, which was only a fancy name for cheese on toast. "Eat up now."

He ate slowly, slicing off pieces and chewing them deliberately between coughs.

She whispered, almost too faint to hear, "Jamesie, it's my birthday today."

"Well, well, isn't that a fine thing! And sure, I've nothing to offer you but a drop of the old uisce beatha for your tea."

"Sure, don't be worrying. I'm just glad for the company." She hesitated and then out it came. "Listen, would you fancy hearing a bit of my novel? I've been writing it ever since I saw you last."

Maher's eyes widened. "You've been busy. I'd be only delighted to listen a while but I'll have to be moving on soon as the engine's running and I'm low on petrol."

Eily brought her jotter down and sat next to her visitor on the settee. She opened the first page and began reading, and it felt to her like leaves winging through the air in autumn, soft and light, each word landing wherever it chose.

Nessa's hair had a raven's hue. It floated in a silken stream down her spine. Her dress was the red of an apple and had been stitched with filaments of spider web. Her voice had the air of flowing water and everyone who heard her was entranced.

Maher's head bowed over his chest, eyes closed, his lips curved in a smile. "Mythic…"

Eily kept reading. *But an angry boy in the town cast a spell on her. He might have been jealous of her kind heart. So now every word she uttered had to be completely true, no matter how it might injure or hurt others. If she told even a fib, a ribbon in her hair would become a knife and slice off a braid.*

Maher groaned in his seat. "Now that's a terrible thing…"

One day, she went to visit the priest in their village to ask his advice about this. His name was Father Lamb.

"Bedad! Isn't that the very name of your own parish priest?"

Eily nodded, not stopping. *But once inside the sacristy, he didn't want to help her, only yanked up her dress from the hem and stuck his fingers into openings in her bottom she had hardly known were there.*

Maher was sitting upright now, staring at Eily. "Now wait…"

Poor Nessa, she was only young and her heart was pure, and she was shocked at the pain and before she could stop herself, she had gone to the toilet all over Father Lamb's hand. His shoes had yellow puddles….

"Oh!" Liam poked his head in the doorway. "Didn't know you were with us, Maher. How's it going?"

Maher cocked his head in Liam's direction, not a word rising out of his mouth.

"Is she annoying you, Maher, with her wild stories? Want me to kick her out?"

Maher pushed himself with force out of the couch and standing tall, said, "No! No, she's grand. You go about your day now. We're content as we are." Liam sauntered off into the kitchen.

Eily opened her mouth to read again. It was like a dam bursting in her throat, the waters of her past gushing out after years of being trapped. Her heart was racing.

Next day, Father Lamb was waiting for her with a cloth in his hand and he told her to bend over.

Maher raised his arm and rocked Eily's shoulder. "That's enough now, Eily."

"I was only warming up."

"Where, may I ask, did you get these stories? It's a wild imagination you have."

Eily looked directly into Maher's tired eyes. "I didn't have to make it up. Nessa speaks only what's true."

Maher sighed long and low. "Would it be all right if I gave you a hug?"

Eily braced herself. *Please God, not him too.*

"It's okay now, child. I only want to thank you for sharing your story with me."

"But there's more."

"I know, I know, and it's gripping, I'll tell you that. But the van's whirring out there and needs a topper upper so I can finish my run."

Eily walked him to the front door and asked, shyly, "Did you like it?"

"Eily, I thought it was a truly amazing story. I'm awed and honored to have heard it. Maybe we can do it in installments, a chapter or two every time I'm here?"

"Sounds brilliant, Jamesie. It'll be like those new shows on telly where they feed you a new piece every week!" Eily was excited, though after her friend left, her stomach tightened. It had felt so good to finally share a little of her secret and yet, she could tell Maher was disturbed by it. The truth seemed to make everyone uneasy whereas a lie slipped out of mouths easy as you like, all foamy spittle and see-through.

On the third day of a house without parents, Liam left Corn Flakes and milk out on the table after him. Eily didn't know was it because he was too lazy to put them away or if he was really thinking of her and left breakfast waiting. It wasn't till she came home from school that she found the note. *Eily, I'd stay out of the house today if I were you. My mates are coming over again.*

It was the first letter she'd received from her brother and she was chuffed. But where would she go? She had homework to do; the end of year exams were coming up soon.

She waited for Kiara after school but there was no sign. Maybe she was sick. On her walk home, Eily took a detour to the Moran's house and rang the bell. It had a loud, sharp sound like teeth grating. At least it worked. The one at Eily's house seemed only for decoration. It was silent as death. She pressed again, a little longer, but no one answered. She knew Kiara's brothers would still be at school at that hour, being older. But where was Mrs. Moran? She was always home. Where was her best friend?

The orange Volkswagen sat in the driveway, a cheery balloon abandoned.

She did jumping jacks on the curb for a while hoping someone, anyone would show up. Eventually she gave up and went home.

As she hunkered down on the back step to do her sums, Eily felt a hand plucking her upwards by the pinched skin on her neck. One minute she was swinging like a rag doll. and the next, she was thrust into the garage, circled by a pack of wild animals.

"Wouldn't she be a looker if she'd a few more years on her?" The ruddy nosed one said.

"More meat, you mean," chipped in the boy with braces.

"Sure, she's only a girl, lads, leave her be." A high-pitched voice from behind. She couldn't see who spoke but the look on the ones she could – vicious, like pit bulls about to pounce – was enough to silence him.

"That uniform doesn't do her any favors, does it, boys?"

"Mammy pressed it only last week," Eily said, proud that the pleats still rested in place, like a brand new accordion.

"Did she now? And what would Mammy say if we were to rip that thing right off you?" Laughs thundering through the thick air. Smoke blowing into her eyes so they watered.

"Ah, she's but a babby, whinging now, she is."

Liam moved forward. She thought he was about to speak up

for her, but his face only puced and he tightened his lips together again.

"I'm thirteen!!"

"Well then, you're old enough to have a puff. A fag'll put hair on you in no time."

She spun her head away from the cigarette, but felt a red hot bee sting through her blouse. No, it was the lit tobacco searing her nipple.

"Would you look at that, lads? A little daisy." Fingers prodding at the fire in her chest.

"Leave off her, lads," Liam's voice echoed from behind Eily. It sounded faint, far off, not the taunting strength she was used to. "Let's just kick her out."

No one seemed to be listening. Eily heard footsteps and the door slam.

"Liam!" She yelled.

"Chicken, chicken," was all she heard, from a voice she didn't recognize, and then, "Lads, let's do it."

She felt herself air lifted onto a wooden stool. From up there, she could smell the red paint on the concrete wall: *Hail Hilter*, it said. She wondered if it was part of a weather forecast. She'd known hail once, great big gobs of ice that'd smack you hard on the head, like Sister Carmelita's leather strap. She enjoyed the feel of it, knowing it was only angel kisses dropping with passion from the heavens. Maybe this too was passion, the wild burning inside her. Though she knew too she'd heard Hitler's name before and that he'd done very bad things to people.

And here she was now, high on her stool, wobbling, taller than any of the snickering boys. They appeared like tin soldiers to her, rusty and dinged. She wanted to show them the rim of light on their shoulders, tell them they didn't have to be so gruff, that God didn't need them to prove a thing.

She thought she saw Liam leave but the rope was descending on her, a rough halo, and the boys were chanting something she couldn't make out, so loud, it almost drowned out her angels, one outshouting the next – "G'on! Chicken, chicken! G'on!" – as the noose trapped her girl neck and grew taut and more taut. Poking from behind at her ribs, her legs. The chair disappeared, a fleet drop. Her cheeks puffed up like balloons from the inside, and a fierce ringing abducted her ears, red thunder shredding her wings, the last vestiges of light leaking out of her until all that remained was black silence.

Hail Hilter! The first thing she saw when she came to. She hadn't noticed before that Hitler was misspelled. Her head was swimming, like someone had dunked her in hot liquid. The back of her skull throbbed. Slowly, she ran her fingers along the jagged ridges on her neck. The whole world seemed to be burning. Her neck felt scorched. And then she noticed the ice of the concrete floor. It was singeing her back.

She was amazed she could move. A baby again learning to walk, she pushed herself up to kneeling. The ceiling seemed to be dancing with the floor. A wisp of twine curled like a snake from her hair. She heard a wild animal screaming, from somewhere far off, so loud it pierced through her ears.

The wall held her steady as she tried to stand, the lasso of rope a rough zero on the ground. Dribbles of blood oozed down her chest. She bent her head, it felt easier than keeping it upright, and skulked out into the cool, clean air.

How long she lay on her bed, who could say? Liam had done a disappearing act. The house was calm for once but inside, Eily was a raging furnace. Teardrops of sweat filmed her face though her skin was cold. She searched through the annals of her brain for a vision of The Face, something, anything to soothe her until she drifted into oblivion.

A bird pecking at the window roused her out of torpor. For

a minute, she wondered where she was, who she was. The black cowl of memory hit then like a hammer at her temples. Slowly, she lurched towards the bathroom. The foggy mirror revealed a girl she hardly recognized, her eyes sharp slits, darkness lurking round her mouth, hair glued to her neck. Dimples of scarlet skin ringed her collarbone. She bathed the blood away with a damp flannel. Hazy. Lost. Nameless.

She was surprised at her appetite. Downstairs, she shoveled handfuls of Rice Krispies into her mouth, though it hurt her throat to swallow, and washed them down with a bottle of milk. It tasted sour but she kept gulping as if it were her last meal on earth. In the cave of her being, she wished it was.

She tore off wedges from the bread loaf and wandered into the sitting room. Empty Smithwicks bottles lined the hearth. The couch was snowed with paper, pages from her novel. She stared at the loose leaves. Someone had torn them out of her jotter. Nessa strewn all over the settee. In an instant, she gathered up the vestiges of her book, clutched them to her chest, then quickly, deliberately tore each one into halves, then quarters, eighths, until a choir of white birds circled her shoes. R.I.P. Nessa of the flowing hair. No more use for her now, no place on this godforsaken earth for truth. Eily wished she could cry but when she searched for her heart, she found only cold, merciless stone.

The angels had fled, and she only had time now for chewing gum and flicking through her mother's old magazines. The sky offered no signs. She left for school in the mornings, the green and yellowing scar on her neck buried under her Aran scarf. Thank God it was cold for summer. No one would question her wearing it but who gave a toss about her anyway? Every time she'd tried to speak about Father Lamb or any of her troubles, she'd been cut off, interrupted, shooed away. And sure, who would she tell? Da was hardly ever home, and Ma, whenever she returned, had big enough worries of her own. What was the point of anything, she wondered. But it only made her head hurt, trying to wrap sense around this unknowable life. She turned right by Miss Doyle's shop and wandered back to the fields, trading her uniform for trousers and a polo neck jumper, and spent hours tossing bread bits at the stupid black cow by the creek.

When her mother finally came home, she was thin, her face the color of chalk. She wouldn't stay in bed and rest like the doctor told her to. Eily found her when she came in from the fields, at the sink, washing dishes. She didn't want to talk about the baby. Or anything. She resembled a gutted, fragile bird, the spirit vacuumed out of her. She had no place to put any more bad news. She told Eily to go upstairs and give her room to make the dinner.

Eily wanted to yell at her to stop moving, to sit and let herself cry. But she could tell how hard her mother was trying to stave off tears. And was she any different herself? She skulked upstairs and played Sandy Shaw on the record player. *Always something there to remind me…*

It wasn't long before she heard her mother's voice. It was raised and brittle. "I will not go, Eamon, and that's final."

"But it's a celebration…" Her father's voice.

"To celebrate what, exactly? We lost the child."

"You'll be blessed by the priest. Surely…"

"No! I do not need to be purified, thank you very much."

Back and forth, like a ping pong ball, they flung arguments at each other. Eily crept down into the hall, her head pounding. "What's going on?"

"Don't blame me if you end up in Purgatory!" Her father slammed the back door behind him.

Eily's mother was sitting on a stool by the sink, rocking back and forth.

"Mum?"

"Your father," there was a bitterness in her voice, "wants me to be Churched."

"What?"

"An outdated ritual." Her mother let out that long sigh that made Eily's skin pucker. "The church – and your father – apparently believe a woman is impure after she's had a baby."

"But you didn't."

A sharp laugh fell out of her mother's mouth. "Ha! Do you think they care! I absolutely refuse to be," she clenched the word in her mouth, *"cleansed* – as if I was dirty by sheer virtue of having a child – cleansed by a priest who has no idea what I've been through. And you know what the bloody irony of it is?" Her mother seemed to be talking to the air.

Eily said nothing.

"You have to pay them for the privilege! Half a crown. Can you imagine?" She was almost spitting with rage. "It's your father should be purified, if truth be told!"

Eily stared, speechless. Did she know about their secret? All these years, Eily had kept her father's nightly visits to herself. It was their special prayer, hadn't he said so himself? And praying was the holiest thing imaginable. Or was it? Heartsick, she wasn't sure of anything these days. Well, he hardly stopped into her bedroom any more anyway, and in some strange way, she almost missed him.

"If Rothman's didn't cost the earth, I'd start smoking again."

Her mother looked at her, as if only now realizing someone was listening, and stood up in a great white heat. "Go Eily, I'm tired. There'll be no more spoken of this. It's done."

When the first blood soaked through her skirts, Eily wasn't afraid. It felt familiar almost, the crimson flood hollowing her body. Liam was the first to spot the ruby puddles in the bathroom. He told her no one would want her now. She thought she'd feel relieved but a bruised cloud hovered over her heart and she understood nothing. Was there anywhere left in the whole wide world where she belonged?

Eily raced out the back door to greet him when she saw the blood dribbling down his neck. No matter how she was feeling, the sight of her father always eased her torments. For all his bluff and banter, she saw beneath to the vulnerable, scared little boy. Like her now, he'd lost his light somewhere in the muddle of days. Who else would take care of him if not her?

"Daddy! What on earth?"

"Ah girl," Her father sighed, his head bowed. He looked almost defeated. "I cycled into a bit of wire."

"How could you do that?"

"I wasn't really thinking." He leaned his bike slowly against the coal house door, dazed. Eily pulled the ironed hanky out of his jacket pocket and gently mopped up the crimson pools ringing her father's throat. It looked like a necklace that appeared and disappeared, a magician's trick.

"Oh Da," she almost pulled her collar down to show him her own scar, a muddle of green and yellow now, in the same place, but stopped herself.

"You'll be better before you're twice married," Eily quoted her mother, doing her best to fight off tears, though maybe they were for herself. He had the look of Jesus on the cross, all wounded and the passion beaten out of him. Her heart cried out for her father, though she said nothing after that, only kept dabbing lightly until the hanky was a wet mess of puce.

EAMON

The headaches had been doing him in for months now, the pressure on his temples like a ten ton lorry. Soon as he got in the back door after work, he'd have to sit down and lower his head into his hands. Hobbled over the kitchen chair, moans rising out of him in a fury he couldn't contain. The constant pounding, how could anyone understand the horror of it, a woodpecker with a beak sharp as glass. And then the voices, Lord help him. All he did was cry out to the heavens for help. And what did he get in return? *You're a failure, a fake father, useless, spent. You'll never amount to anything.* On and on they ranted with their drivel. *You're a goner, Purgatory's too good for you. You'll pay for your sins.*

And visions then, the heft of Jack behind him, ramming his thick wedge into his backside. Flashes of blue lightning streaking through him. The clouds a scum of gray making a mist of him. "What's so special down there in the grass, lad? Let me show you something you'll really like."

And he bloody and sore after, longing to kick the shite out of that bastard. But all he could do, then and now, was fold into himself and pull a curtain over the black pictures ruining his brain.

Night after night without sleeping a wink, it was too much for him. Even the girl couldn't pull him out of it though she wanted to, she did. She'd rub his hands warm when he came in the door, make scalding tea for him in his favorite mug. But he'd lost heart somewhere in all this chaos. Too many thoughts scourging him that just wouldn't stop. One after another, they piled up in a slag heap. His head on fire. That Casey at work. He had it in for him, he did, he knew it from the start. Couldn't look at him without a mean comment gushing out of his dirty mouth. *How's it going, Eamon? Needing any help, Eamon? Would you like me to double check this for you, Eamon?* As if he meant a word of it. It was him, no doubt about it, ringing all the time and when he'd pick up the phone, only silence. Taunting him, Casey was, the messer. Next thing, he'd be breaking into the house, taking every last thing he cherished.

Well, he'd see about that, wouldn't he? The world may be out to get him but he was tough, he'd survived the horror this long, hadn't he? Yes, he'd put a stop to it. He put a double bolt on the back door and a padlock over that. Only he had the code, that'd show them. And a pile of chairs wedged against the latch. Just let anyone try to break down that.

For a minute, he'd feel a little ease until the panic rose up in flames again. He even went after the girl, grabbed her from behind when she was in the toilet but he was cold inside, couldn't get his fire going.

"Daddy?"

Couldn't even speak. Tears dripping out of his eyes, he slumped into his bed and shook, a limp grass scoured by the wind.

"I'll get it!" The phone was so loud, he thought it'd split his ears in two. "Let me get it." Tearing into the dining room, he nearly knocked the phone over, lunging for the receiver.

Only a buzz when he lifted the ear piece. "I knew it! I knew it, Mother! He's out to get me, d'ye hear, he wants me dead."

"Eamon," his wife standing above him, like a stone statue. "There's no one there. Can't you see? The phone never rang."

"Are you mad, woman? It rang so loud it nearly took the head off me!"

"No Eamon, I'm sorry. You must have been imagining it. I was right here and heard nothing."

"Well, maybe you need a hearing aid then."

So she was in on it too, God help him, pretending he'd made it all up. Who could he trust any more? Even his own family after him now.

"You pick it up next time, why don't you, and then you'll see," he struggled out of the chair.

"I will when it rings, Eamon."

He shoved her arms away. "Get off me, woman. You're no better than Casey himself."

How was a man to rest when he'd a storm of people trying to break him? Who could he turn to? Even God wasn't listening, only adding to the jeers in his head. He stumbled up the stairs, his armpits drenched in sweat.

She was sitting on the lower bunk bed when he came in.

"Daddy? What's wrong?"

He grabbed the girl's dress again, tried to ruch it up. Where had he gone? Lord have mercy on him, helpless he was and he needing help more than ever.

And then the stupid wire. He hadn't seen it, so many thoughts hammering at his forehead. The gouges in his neck, blood spurting everywhere. He'd wheeled the bike slowly home. It was too big a cross to bear, no man should have to carry it.

If only herself hadn't come out and caught the girl dabbing him clean. If only she'd waited five more minutes, she mightn't have noticed.

"That's it, Eamon. You need help."

"Sure, I'm grand, can't you see it's just a bit of blood?"

"I've suspected something wrong for a long time and this is the final straw."

"But…"

"No buts, Eamon. I'm making the call."

And that would be that. The men in white coats come to take him away to some miserable place where he could rot in Hell. Well, it couldn't be any worse than this.

"Mammy, what call are you on about?"

"Your father needs to rest, Eileen. He's been overtaxed for a long time now. Don't you worry. He'll be well taken care of. Thank God we're insured."

She marched into the house like a soldier who is set firm on his mission, a smell of scorched skin in her wake.

EILY

"Oh, it's you, Jamesie." From the front stoop, Eily watched old Maher shuffle up the path.

"I took a detour on my route cos I'm wanting to hear more of your book, girl."

Eily lowered her eyes. "Too late." Her voice sharper than she intended. Maher meant well, she knew.

"Why's that?"

"Tore it up, it was stupid, anyway."

"You didn't! Oh Eily."

Silence.

He rested his hip against the front wall. "Is it your father?" His voice soft. "Shame about what happened to him. He was the best footballer in Drogheda, before he became a rugby star, that is. Famous he was, in our parish."

"Nothing happened," Eily said firmly as she could. "He was tired, is all."

"Ah now…"

Maher put a clumsy arm around Eily's shoulder. "There, there, girl."

"It's no use anymore," her voice quivering. "Just no use." And then the tears erupted, like an army that had been waiting for the word to advance.

The comfort of Maher's embrace, his gentleness, and Eily couldn't contain her sorrows any longer. "The garage… boys… a rope," on and on her tale of woes spilled out onto the waiting air.

She felt the old man stiffen but he held her steady as her body shook. "Now, now. It's all going to turn out right. Cross my heart."

The telephone ringing was a jagged breach in their communion. "I need to answer that," Eily patted down her uniform and stood up. "Have to go."

Maher fell backwards as Eily moved away. He raised his cap to her, bowing slightly. "I'll be back, girl. You can be assured of that."

It was almost dark when Eily closed the front gate behind her. She had to get out of that lonely house, wander the fields a while, erase the images of her father strapped to a bed in St. John of God's, of all the stories she had emptied into her weary friend. She felt raw inside, like a wound had been pierced and was seeping pus again.

As she turned onto Ballygall Road, she was surprised to see Kiara leaning against McLoughlin's wall, a cigarette dangling out of her mouth. "You scared the life out of me!"

Kiara laughed, a harshness in her throat.

"Where've you been? I went round to your place a load of times looking for you."

"Had to see a man about a dog," she took a long drag and blew swirls of smoke out into the gloaming. "Nah, my ma took me on the train to visit Auntie Rosie in Sligo."

"In the middle of school?"

Kiara looked harder somehow, not the light-hearted friend she'd grown to love only a few weeks ago. But everything was changing, even for her.

"Yeah, well…" She didn't want to talk about it, just shrugged her shoulders. "How's tricks with you, then?"

For a second, Eily considered telling her about the night in the garage, about her father's breakdown, about not going to school, but she was tired from all she'd shared with Maher and from the looks of it, Kiara had worries of her own. They stood together in the wordless air until Kiara held out the stub of her Sweet Afton and Eily waved it away.

The lads always seemed to be hanging around. It was all Kiara wanted to do since she'd come home, sit on the wall with them and slag each other and chew gum. Declan Arnold had a thing for Eily's hair. "Toss it back again, will ye? It looks like flames in the air." Eily dipped her hair down and flicked it back over her head a few times but got tired of it. When Declan gave her a charm that said Love on it, she dropped it on the ground and legged it home. Kiara shouted after her but she kept going.

On Valentine's Day, Declan came to her door with a card. "I'm giving you one so you should give me one back." Eily opened the card. It had old-fashioned roses on the front and inside a drawing of a girl with her hair on fire. *That's you,* it said. And next to it, a smiling boy with glasses on, reaching for the girl's hand. *Me!*

Eily closed the door on him and went straight for her mother's purse. She wasn't used to the new money yet – it was all decimals and pence – but grabbed a bill and took off down the road to Vincent's Hair Shop. It was a little shed on the side of a house in Tolka Estate. Eily waited her turn and finally, Vincent sat her in the big chair and asked what style she was after.

"Chop it off, please." Eily announced. She walked home, a chill on her bare neck, smiling, light as a bird.

Kiara stopped waiting for her after school. Eily would catch a glance of her on Cremore wrapped round a lad she didn't know. He looked old. Kiara'd pull out from under him to wave sometimes but they hadn't passed words in a long while. Declan Arnold wouldn't look at her. And all Leeper could offer was, *Who loves ya, baby?* Or, *howaya, Kojak.*

One afternoon, she went home the long way. A work crew was drilling on her road. The lid was off the man hole. Eily moved around it. An older man with a gap in his teeth whistled after her, *Pretty woman, walkin' down the street.* Eily spun round on her heels, took one hard look at him, and launched a wad of spit that landed on his left boot.

When she came through the back door, there he was. Her father slumped over the kitchen table, his head wedged between his hands.

"Da!" She shrieked. "You're home!"

Eily moved to embrace him but one of his elbows slid off the table and she ended up kissing the crown of his head.

"You look tired. I thought you were supposed to be resting."

"Ah girl, I suppose I did but sure, the weariness keeps on mounting, doesn't it? It's like a tap that never turns off."

He was all wrapped into himself, didn't even notice her hair. What use had the doctors been when he was only a rag doll. She liked him better full of guff and bluster.

"I've a surprise for you. Look in the breakfast room."

Eily tip toed into the adjoining room and found a small stool with bands of all colors interwoven across the seat.

"I made it myself with my very own hands."

It was bright as summer. Eily stared, mesmerized, imagining the dark corners of her father's heart swimming away from him with each movement of his hands. She could hardly imagine his hulking fingers conjuring something so delicate.

"It's a beauty," she lifted the stool up and spun it around.

"Why don't you sit on it, girl? It's more sturdy than it looks."

Eily could tell how pleased her father was with his creation as she plopped down on it, the colored straps swaying beneath her. Swinging on a rainbow. She was so proud of him, she thought her heart would break. It was faint but the singing started up again inside her. Some things, not many, were still right with the world.

After that he took to wandering the roads. She'd find him some evenings on the avenue, bent over like a humbled monk, huffing. His stiff arms would be groping for twigs tossed from hedges and trees in the March winds. She wanted to shout, "Da! Can I help?" But he was on his own mission so she let him be. He'd pile up his stash on the footpath, as if he were going to light a fire there, and then hoosh the lot over his shoulder, and on he'd shuffle home, nose dripping, Dick Whittington content with his bounty.

When he finally went back to work, Eily would wait near the back door until night opened its arms over the bleak town. She could feel the bitter chill through the cracks in the window. He'd be huffing his way up the Washerwoman's Hill now on his bicycle, rain pelting him in the face, his thinning gloves no match for the north wind. The strength of those rugby days long leaked out of him, and he only halfway up and knackered. Off to the side of the road then, and hoist one leg over the bar.

He'd push a path home, him and his bike, he'd get there no matter what, for he knew, he surely knew, didn't he, that she'd be waiting there, rubbing her palms together to toast his. And the clink of the loose chain on his bike would tell her he was coming round the coal house now, almost there, and she'd swing open the door, arms launched towards him.

"Let me take that for you, Da," and she'd lean the bike against the garage door. "In you come to the warmth."

And he'd have hardly a foot in the door before she'd start into their favorite poem. *When icicles hang by the wall, and Dick the shepherd blows his nail* and he'd pick it up, *And Tom bears logs into the hall, and milk comes frozen home in pail.* And she pulling the soaked hanky from his breast pocket, not missing a beat, he dripping all over her, they'd skip to their favorite line, singing together, *And Marion's nose is red and raw...* And then, almost children again, they'd whisper the line her mother hated, *Tu-whit, to-whoo, a merry note, While greasy Joan doth keel the pot,* she all the while cosseting his frozen fingers with her hands, rubbing the chill, the long, bad day, all heartache far away.

Each June, his old boarding school, Castleknock, would have a Summer Fête, and he, the old sports hero, would be invited. Eily was proud of him, winning all those caps for Ireland in his rugby days. She didn't care that he traded his free passes to Landsowne for anti-depressants. Sure hadn't she many's the time taken the 19 across town all the way to Rialto, the terminus on the south side, to pick up his prescriptions? But no one could take away those glory days, there were photos, clippings from the Irish Times and the Independent and Evening Herald of that muscled second row forward. People used to chase him down Abbey Street for an autograph.

He never wanted to talk about it, let the matches come and go, he said, let Doctor Riordan watch them from the stands where he could have been. Sure what was the use anyway? But Eily kept the memory fresh in her heart and conjured it when she felt he needed cheering.

She elected to go with him to Castleknock. Though it was rarely mentioned, Uncle Jack had paid for his first year at the fancy school with his boxing winnings. After that, he didn't need to for her father got a full scholarship on account of his sporting prowess.

Three buses, and a long walk to reach those gray iron gates. He wore a suit nearly the same shade, faded, and a striped tie. Eily took his hand and he carried his huge umbrella in the other.

Eily wasn't sure what she'd expected, maybe those rich politicians and doctors fawning over her father's triumphs on the pitch. Instead, she listened, time and again, as the men in their blazers bearing the school crest, shook her father's hand.

"Ah, Eamon. How are you keeping these days? Looking well."

And her father with his hand in theirs, gripping like it was the last hand on earth he'd ever touch. She wanted to wrench each poor man's hand's free but stood one foot on top of the other to quiet herself.

To the police superintendent, he said, "This is my daughter, Eily."

"Grand girl she is… Have you any boys?"

"Just the one, Officer. We'd a second but he didn't make it."

And to the T.D. from County Meath and everyone else who posed the same question, "Is your lad at school here?"

"Ah no, Simon, no. We're too poor."

Eily would wince at each man's embarrassment, scarlet inside, and try to urge her father onwards.

"Why d'you have to tell them that, Da?"

"Sure it's true, isn't it? It's the gospel truth."

It may have been so, bills piling up, income dwindling, but all the same, he insisted on flagging down a taxi on their way out. "We might be going downhill, Eily," he slid his arm inside hers as they walked towards the waiting car, like two school pals, "but we'll surely go down in style!"

At first she thought she was imagining it, but every time she turned around, the boy was half a block behind her. He'd stall, look into a garden, scratch his head, open his satchel, and yet he never lost that few feet between them. Finally, she cornered him.

"Why are you hanging round? Who are you?"

"Tristan," he said, his face melting into a shy smile.

"Well, what are you after, Tristan?"

"I go to St. Vincent's in Phibsboro. I know your father, Eamon, from First Fridays at the church."

A light flashed in Eily's head. She'd been about to correct the boy, tell him to call her father Mr., but no, she'd call him Eamon too. It'd be almost as if he was her pal. Or even her boyfriend. That'd keep the young messers away.

"Do you, now? Well, Eamon told me only yesterday not to talk to strangers." It wasn't true but now that Nessa was dead, what room was there for truth? No one paid it a bit of heed, anyway.

"I'm not really a stranger. I played soccer with your brother once."

Eily flinched at the mention of Liam. "Soccer? Eamon was a famous rugby player, did you know that? Played for Ireland, won a load of caps, they're on our sitting room wall." On and on she went, delighted with her new plan, her new boyfriend. There'd always been a special bond between her father, those times in her bedroom, though she could hardly conjure what had happened there. Using his first name would make them closer again. "Eamon took me to his old boarding school for the summer Fête…"

The boy listened, carefully.

"Good on him," he said. "But listen, "I was wondering more about you, you know, if you'd…"

"Spit it out, Tristan, if I'd what?" She had little patience for boys these days. It was all the girls in school were interested in, always putting on their sister's make up and waiting for them to pass by. And then they'd shout out stupid things and make eejits of themselves. Eily couldn't be bothered. Couldn't they see the lads were all the same, gawky, angry teenagers trying too hard to prove themselves?

Somehow Tristan seemed different, though, softer, gentle. His sideways smile lit up his face as he switched his copy book from one hand to the other.

"Would you want to maybe go out with me?"

"Are you chancing your arm?"

"We wouldn't have to do much, just take a walk together or something."

Eily didn't know what to say.

"What's in your jotter?"

"I'm just after finishing art class. It's only a few drawings."

"Here, show me," Eily grabbed the book from under his arm and skimmed through the pages. "That's a nice dandelion." She said, remembering how she used to love the flowers in O'Reilly's garden.

"You really like it?" Tristan was all lit up.

"And a girl! What are you drawing girls for, for God's sake?"

"I'm practicing so I can draw you."

"Some day, Eamon's going to do my portrait." Eily was surprised at how easily the lies piled up.

She leaned with him against the railings of a big house and let the boy talk, though he wasn't really a boy, but a young man.

He said he'd seen her walking the avenue, always alone, how he'd wanted to take her hand and kiss her sadnesses away. His voice didn't have that brittle edge to it, only warmth, and if she admitted it, kindness. It was almost tea time when she said she'd better go.

"Can we chat another time?"

Eily wasn't sure if she liked him or hated him. She shrugged.

As soon as she got in the back door, Eily cornered her father who was leaning over insurance papers at the kitchen table. "Eamon..." she whispered.

"Mmm?" Her father didn't look up.

"Eamon." She drew in a long breath. "I've started calling you Eamon, you know, out on the street. What d'you think about that? Eamon?"

"Grand, Eily," her father scratched his temple. "Whatever you say. I'm occupied here. These bloody quarterly reports..."

Eily didn't need any more, and sidled upstairs to her bedroom, content with her new found partner. She put on her favorite LP, *Stand By Me*.

Next morning, her father was waiting for her in the hallway when she came down for breakfast. "Ah, if it isn't Eamon!" Eily had a bounce to her voice. "How's my old pal doing this fine day?"

"Eily," her father's voice sounded stern. "I've been thinking."

"About what, Eamon?"

"Don't!" He said, sharply. "Just don't!"

"What, Eamon?"

"Eileen," he placed a hand on the edge of her shoulder. "I don't want you calling me Eamon any more. I'm your father and the only father you'll ever have."

"But Eamon..."

"Stop now, Eily. I've had enough. It's a sacred relationship, father and child, and you need to respect it."

Eily opened her mouth to speak but her father intercepted. "No more nonsense, girl. Daddy it is, from now on. If you don't like it, find somewhere else to live."

Eily stood a moment, the shock holding her in place, her chance to show off her closeness to someone, especially her father, leaking out the hole in her heart. Eventually, she sidled back upstairs and slammed the door to her room.

The following afternoon, Tristan was sitting with his pals beyond the convent gate when Eily came out. He jumped off the wall and almost ran towards her. The lads were taunting him but he didn't seem to be listening.

He walked her home that afternoon and the next and the next until the weekend came. Tristan's company eased the sorrow inside her, even her father pushing her away now. Where did she belong anymore? It wasn't just boys, Eily thought, girls too. There was no one in her world she could depend on.

Tristan, on the other hand, didn't fall into either category. He was easy in his skin, and always happy to see her. And he didn't tell her what to do, just accepted her for who she was. He made her laugh more than once. The muscles in her jaw slowly softened but the cramping in her chest never seemed to ease up.

"When can I see you again?"

"Sunday," the words came out before she could shove them back down. "I'll be at the Botanics about 4."

"Great! I live just round the corner from there."

On Saturday, Eily's mother came home with a bag full of shopping. "I ran into Mrs. Moran up at Whitty's." She took the groceries out of her bag. "It seems that Kiara has gone."

Eily looked up from her magazine. "Gone where?"

"That I don't know, dear. Her parents decided she'd be better off schooled elsewhere, away from the rougher elements. Somewhere in the country, I believe. She's staying with an aunt."

Eily slammed the tea pot on the table. She hadn't seen Kiara for weeks but still, she had been her closest friend. Why hadn't she told her she was leaving?

"I'm going out, Ma," Eily grabbed her coat from the breakfast room.

"Mum!"

"Yeah, yeah," Eily muttered as she went out into the fierce wind, letting it blow her wherever it chose. If she wanted someone to rely on, she realized, it would have to be herself. A wave of determination washed through her. Forget the lot of them, she decided, as she came to the end of her road. Miss Doyle's shop had been demolished. The men in yellow macintoshes were busy building new houses. Soon there'd not even be a patch of field left for her to wander in. She climbed over the fence and past the big sign that said, *No Trespassing*. On she trudged, kicking dented Cidona cans out of the way.

He was sitting under the last remaining tree, tossing sticks in the air. "Declan, what're you doing here?"

"Passing time till me ma gets home." His face was drooping on one side. "The house is locked while she's at work."

There was a pink tinge to his cheeks. Eily wondered if he was embarrassed. They'd not spoken a word since she'd slammed the door on his Valentine card.

"She works on Saturdays?"

He nodded. "Doesn't matter what day it is, people need their houses cleaned."

Eily sighed. There was so much you couldn't ever predict in this world and yet some things droned on in the same boring way day after day. She sat down next to him. "Kiara's away. Did you know that?"

He shook his head. "Last I saw her, she was with Gerry, that older bloke, you know, from Finglas? He hung around with us for a while but I think he got bored."

"Well, she's off down the country now."

"Eily, I don't suppose you've changed your mind about me?"

"You suppose right."

"Just one small date? I promise, I'll be good."

Eily wondered if he wasn't so much interested in her but in having a girlfriend. A light flickered inside her. "Tell you what. I'll meet you at the Botanics tomorrow about 4. Okay?"

Declan's eyes opened so wide, they looked like they'd knock his glasses off. "Ye will?"

"Yeah," Eily felt a thin, dark rope pull taut inside her. "I will."

She wandered home slowly, a tight smile on her lips.

On Sunday afternoon, the rains were lashing. Two o'clock. Half past three. Four. She ran a bath upstairs, locked the door, and watched wisps of her hair float on the surface like sparks.

Not two weeks had passed when Maher showed up again. Eily was sitting on the front stoop watching the leaves spiral through the air. "Jamesie." Much as she liked him, she couldn't seem to muster much feeling about anything. "Did we order kerosene again?"

Old Maher had a glint in his eye. "That's not why I'm here, Eily." He smiled so wide that she saw the tobacco stains on his back teeth. "I've been having a wild notion."

He said seeing as her father wasn't so well and her mother either and besides, she herself seemed to be mitching from school, well, she was already a truant. What future did she have here? Far be it from him to change her life, but just in case she'd have interest, he'd had a brainwave.

Why not live with him and be his housekeeper, sure, she mightn't even pass the Leaving Cert and she'd not get another job with half the country unemployed. He had a house in Annagassan, he said, that needed attention.

Eily thought he was jousting with her.

"I've a little put away. It wouldn't be much but I could pay you each week and you'd have your own room and all the Welsh Rarebits you can stomach."

Maher leaned towards her, keeping her gaze, a man on a mission. "I'll leave you to consider it, Eily. Either way, you'll still be my dear friend."

Eily stared after him, stunned. His dear friend, he'd called her. Dear. Friend.

Only friend. Her heart was beating fast as she went back inside.

Next time he came, Maher slid an envelope into Eily's hand. A cashier's check lay inside the folds of a short letter. She stared at it as if it were a new species of animal, holding it up to the light like she'd seen bank clerks do to see if it was real. She studied it as if it held the answer to all her problems.

Eily,

You're a topper of a girl. Young woman, really. And I only want the best for you. It worries me a bit that you're not so happy there at home. Now I don't have much to offer you myself, I know that, but it'd be my pleasure to share it with you. Only if you want.

Best wishes,
your friend Jamesie

Now her father was back at work, he stayed long hours at the office. And her mother, well, she still put meals on the table but barely spoke two words to Eily any more. Lost in her own world of sorrows, she was. Yet how could she leave them, these two creatures who seemed more lost than even she was? She felt a tear in her heart. Longing to protect her wounded father, her fragile mother, keep them safe. And then an opposite tug inside her, to find her own way – she was almost fifteen after all – to be free of the dark shadows clouding the house.

As she sat on the couch, her head glutted with questions, the back door slammed.

"Ma! You here?"

Liam found her in the sitting room. "There she is," he shouted through the doorway. "Doing nothing, as usual."

Eily could feel the heat rise in her. "Who're you to talk? What did you ever do to help anyone?"

"What're you on about?" Liam was pulling gum out of the wrapper.

"Leaving me for dead with your so-called pals."

"You survived, didn't you? I told you to steer clear of my mates, didn't I? And anyway, you don't look any worse for wear."

She wouldn't show him, give him the satisfaction of knowing how hard it had been on her. "You haven't a clue!" she yelled.

"No, it's you haven't an iota! Bet you didn't know that it was me had Terry put down."

Eily couldn't breathe.

"Yeah," her brother tossed the white stick of gum in his mouth, chewing out the side. "Timmons went round complaining to all the neighbors who had dogs. Said they were chasing his sheep. No one could be bothered listening. But I," he spat the gum into the fire. "I talked to Da, convinced him Terry was the problem."

Eily's knees buckled as she tried to stand up. "You didn't."

"Of course, it wasn't the dog was the problem, really. It was always you."

The noise in Eily's head made her dizzy. It wasn't angels or even God. It was a black glob of hysteria. Before she could speak, Liam had gone, the door banging behind him. She sat motionless but for her body wracking, until the day washed away.

By nightfall, she had slipped the cashier's check under her blouse as she crawled into her bed for the final time.

Maher picked her up on the corner of Cremore Road in his Morris Minor. He'd left his van at home, he said. For a moment, she wondered if he'd veer off down a back alley but he just ruffled her hair lightly, like you'd pet a favored animal, and they were off.

The cottage in Annagassan was small and whispered of loneliness. It felt like no one had opened the blinds for years to let the light in. It sat on a large wedge of land and looked out onto a tapestry of fields. Standing on the front stoop, Eily's eyes feasted on the varied shades of green, exhaling long and loud. It was as if all those luscious words for green she'd dreamed up back in primary school had finally come to life. Not even a mile away, her father had grown up. She tried to imagine him as a boy tramping the fields with his pals, unearthing birds' nests. She'd have to take care not to run into Aunt Lily or she'd be in hot water.

Eily got to work dusting, sweeping, washing dishes. She even had Maher hold a ladder for her so she could clean the upstairs windows until they sparkled. Her mother had never let her help in the house, not trusting her to do anything as well as she herself could. Eily was chuffed to see she had it in her, the ability to create a handsome home.

She liked the routine of this new life, Maher lighting the fire in the mornings before he took off on his rounds while she stitched some sheets together to make curtains. In the afternoons, she'd put on Maher's wellies, squelching around the fields in them, drinking in the bird song. Smell of cows in the distance. Wild cats scurrying through the hedgerows. She could breathe here, out in the open, no houses or buildings to hem her in.

In the evenings, she'd fry eggs and rashers for Maher's supper, leaving his slippers by the front door for when he'd come home again. She loved being able to make a difference in someone's life, being useful. The old man would always make a big fuss over his food, though it was simple enough. "Bedad, you're a grand cook, Eily. Can't remember the last time I came home to the smell of a fry and a warm house."

After they'd eaten, Maher would pour himself a snifter of brandy and they'd pull their chairs close to the hearth, staring into the bright flames. Sometimes Eily would read to him from the Treasury Of Irish Poetry she'd found in the cellar. *Once more the storm is howling and half hid under this cradle-hood, my child sleeps on.* His head would bob, and Eily would lift the glass from him and tuck a blanket across his lap.

Once when he'd been half asleep, she'd put his limp arm around her shoulders and dragged him to his bed. Eily knew it was better for his chest if he slept lying down. Once settled under the covers, he'd opened his eyes a little, raised his hand. When he touched her, it was only to stroke an oily, grateful finger down her arm.

Other evenings, they'd stay at the table, leaning over the dirty plates and share stories. He'd been married once, for a year or so before his wife took off with the postman. "Bad cess to her," he grumbled into his soup. "She didn't deserve me."

"No, she didn't." And she thought of Tristan, who'd been kind to her and how she'd left him waiting at the Botanics and how Declan would have waited too in the rain, all hopeful and full of expectation. She felt a stab in her heart. She knew well the sadness of being left alone. Why had she done it? One day maybe, she'd write to Tristan, tell him how sorry she was, that he, like Maher, deserved better. And maybe Declan too.

Occasionally she thought about ringing home to say where she was. But who'd care anyway? No, this was her new life. She could be whoever she wanted. She could let the torment of the past wash away on the tide. Maybe she'd find that open, trusting person she used to be again some day.

With her allowance, Eily saved up for twelve months to buy an old Cortina. She'd almost reached the legal driving age for a provisional license. At Christmas, she and Maher had gone shopping together. A farmer up in Dunleer had no use for his car any more. The muffler had worn out and it made a loud, popping sound as Eily watched Maher steer it out of the drive. But oh, it was lovely, even the faded green and the dented bumper. To Eily, it whispered of freedom.

Maher taught her how to engage the gears, how and when to brake. She took to it, a moth to flame, driving the back roads for hours, while Maher was off on his rounds. The blackberry thickets along the byways seemed to sing her name. She savored the sting of thorns piercing her skin raw.

And long, ragged lines of poetry, taken to heart from Maher's tattered Treasury. She'd pull over next to a field, share the words with passing birds, with the willows in the marsh, with herself. *And for an hour I have walked and prayed because of the great gloom that was in my mind.*

That old Yeats knew about the torments of life, she wagered, glad she had a companion in words, long buried though he was.

One afternoon, she found herself in Drogheda town and on a whim, went into Spar to get Maher's favorite beer. He often liked a sup before he hung up his hat. Eily marveled at how, at sixteen, she could buy alcohol but only have a provisional license to drive.

"Young Eileen, by God, is that yourself?"

Eily turned quickly to find Mrs. Whitty with eyes wide as capital Os staring at her. "Who else would it be?"

"Tsk," Mrs. Whitty puckered her lips. "Sure, isn't your mam and da sick with worry over you?"

Something caught in Eily's throat and she coughed. "Listen, I'm taking care of myself now." Her voice stern as she could make it.

Mrs. Whitty stared.

"And what are you doing up here, anyway?"

"The husband gets some provisions from these parts. I'm just picking the last box of fresh eggs to take home…. Listen, have you a word for your mammy I can pass along?"

Eily hesitated. "Say nothing, please, and I'll give them a ring in the morning, let them know I'm all right."

The woman seemed to get her strength back. "I heard tell you missed your final exams. What'll the nuns say?"

"Not a word, Mrs. Whitty, please. Now if you'll excuse me…"

She watched herself being watched as she paid for the two bottles of lager and left.

Eily's mother was hysterical on the phone when she rang. "I hired a taxi and looked all over Dublin for you."

"I'm not in Dublin anymore, actually."

"I'm well aware of that, Eileen. Mr. Maher at least had the decency to write us and tell us your whereabouts."

"He did?"

"And good thing he did or we'd have gone to the Police. How did I raise such a recalcitrant child?"

"I'm not a child, Ma, and I'm sorry…"

"Is that all you have to say to me… Ma?"

"Sorry, I suppose, but I've found a new life now and I'm happy and sure, you're better off without me."

Her mother said nothing.

"Well, aren't you?"

"Your father said he was going to get you a cake with as many candles on it as days you were away."

Eily laughed though she was touched. "It'd have to be a massive cake for the months I've been gone already."

She wondered if her mother had shed even a tear for her. The line buzzed between them like empty air. "Tell him thanks for the thought. And you for looking out for me. But you can't say you miss me now, can you?"

Silence.

Her heart skipping. Eily put down the phone.

One morning, Eily took Maher in his tea and toast but he was on the floor, eyes sunken into their sockets, the balls like white stones not of this world. The tray crashed to the floor as she knelt beside him. His hand cold as March. Nothing left of him but a shell and still the avalanche of tears, her whole body retching. Tears for her loyal friend at first, then for herself.

Days rose and fell before she got up again. Picking her way through the shattered porcelain, kicking past the tea pot, she put on her winter coat and got in the car.

The wind had the trees rocking. Not a bird for miles. She let the wheel steer her forward, not caring where she went. And then she saw them. A glut of sheep wedged tight between the posts of a gate and a farmer with his cane, flailing at their rumps. Before she knew it, she had veered off the road and in no time, her foot pressed hard on the gas pedal, the whole landscape speeding up as in a dream, she rammed full force into the fold. A fierce thud as four legs ricocheted off the roof of the car. Wild bleating like a song she'd long forgotten, sheep falling all around her, until she could move no further, only stare at the blood weeping down the windscreen.

She had to climb over the gear stick to get out the passenger door. Tripping over a seeping carcass, she picked herself up slowly. A man's voice thundering through the air. Not looking behind her, she ran on through the field and over the hillock until she came to a pond thick with geese droppings. She shed her heavy coat, boots, unleashed her hair, and waded into the icy liquid. Watching the bubbles of crimson flower around her, she lowered herself into the delicious purity of water making room just for her.

It was dusk before she waded out, blue and shivering like she would when Father Lamb first poked at her. But now she felt light, a feather having traveled a great distance, almost like air, as her bare feet carried her towards the trees. And oh, in the gloaming, she couldn't be imagining it, surely, surely, there was a glimmer – she floated cautiously towards it – of that Face, that perfect light – if she could only get there – just around the next bend.

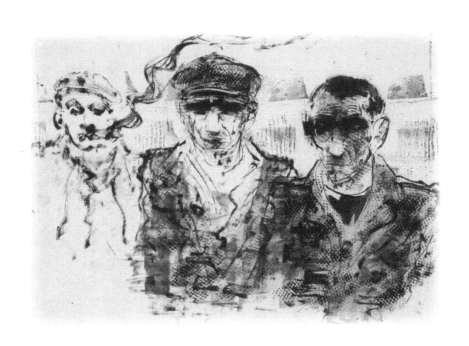

Book 2

THE OREGON TRAIL

…and memory itself
has become an emigrant,
wandering in a place
where love dissembles itself as landscape

– Eavan Boland

It was the sky that shocked you. You'd never seen such a vast, open canvas stretching without end, like a book you'd never finish. It seemed so far away, so unlike the glutted clouds hovering over Ireland, hemming you into your small diocese, holding you in place as that tiny pinpoint on a map, a forgotten membrane. You'd been afraid at first. Who would have thought a place that speaks the same language would feel entirely different?

And those trees, endless flourishes of emerald spiring up to the heavens as if they knew the secret to the universe. You remember being driven from the airport down long, straight rows of streets, and how each house had its own unique flavor. Colors galore. An embarrassment of shades to feast on.

But that was twenty years ago. Oregon dissolved at some point into a replica of Ireland – cool, dark winters and excessively generous rain. You missed the soft rises of Louth, where you could race up and down in almost a single breath. Of course, there were the Dublin mountains out in Wicklow. You'd had a sliver of a glimpse of them from your mother's bedroom window. A swath of mossy green between two chimneys across the road. Da would stand there ogling and chant his anthem. "Sure, we've a tip top view of the mountains from home. Why bother going there?" Here Mount Hood seemed to have fallen from the sky, a majestic edifice in cream and cinnamon that would take days and equipment to mount.

You were lucky, though. You'd had London as a bridge, a window into the widening world. It was a miracle you found the chambermaid's job at the Ritz Carlton, just when you needed it. The darkness after Jamesie died, the caul of bitterness shrouding your every move, and the horror of those mutilated sheep in your wake. Days of lying on the floor next to Jamesie's corpse, fingers entwined, wishing to follow him into the abyss, to be freed of the relentless tug of gravity. But the smell was too much eventually, even for you, as decay set in.

You hid behind the large oak at the cemetery, watching the few mourners pass, a blur of crows. Once the prayers had been said and the last sod of earth tossed over his coffin, you slunk out of hiding and threw yourself onto the earth, wanting to claw it off your best friend in the world. But he wasn't your friend anymore, was he? All that you'd loved, every last shred, was dead and buried. You might as well do the same with the past, inter it in the secret chambers of your battered heart. Sure, what was the use of it any more?

So the ad in the Dunleer Post was a godsend. Room and board, airfare paid, and a workable wage at the London Ritz. You piled your entire belongings into two Penneys shopping bags and hitched a lift in a lorry that wheezed like a dying animal and were dropped off at the Hole-In-The-Wall pub. You'd had to leg it, trailing your carrier bags along the airport road. If you missed the flight, you'd be done for, the hotel was picking up the tab. You lashed through the revolving doors and ran to the end of the queue. But it was long. You'd never make it with all these holidaymakers waiting to check in. So you shuffled up front. An American in a bright green tee shirt that read *Erin Go Bragh* was first in line.

"Sir, I'm terrible sorry," you said to him, "but my plane's about to take off. Could I ever slip in ahead of you?"

He'd looked you up and down, took in the plastic bags and his mouth turned up like a crescent moon. Oh God, those teeth were virgin white. "Go for it!" He nudged you, not aware of his strength, ahead of him. Go for it! He'd said, as if all you had to do in this world was believe you could and so it was. You nodded at him in appreciation and slapped your ticket on the counter and got to the plane just as they were making their final call.

Go for it! It sounded so positive, so Can Do, so far from the 'don't look half sideways at anything, sure, ye'll amount to nothing'

Irish children were spoonfed. America was the land of plenty. Opportunity. New beginnings. Self-made women and men. Sure, you could become anything over there, with a little grit and determination. You liked the openness of Americans, the way they weren't a bit shy. Those three magic words rang in your heart the whole way across the channel. Yes, you would go for it, as soon as you could.

London blurred over time, hazy months of bed-changing, cleaning up spilled whiskey, eating potato pellets in the cafeteria, the alluring scent of burgers grilling in cafes as you walked home to your miniature bedsit. You stayed busy, trying to ignore the shaking arms as visions of sheep flying, bleeding, dying, crowded your thoughts.

You'd been too numb to find the farmer, to explain, apologize. But the ghosts of that day hovered over you, siphoning off your sleep, until you became almost a machine, wiping toilets and bathtubs on automatic. Even as your limbs shivered and slowed, your mind seemed to speed up in equal measure. It became a wild and tortured creature you couldn't control.

Barely able to shuffle up High Street in the dawn light, you were given a warning at work. If they dropped your wages, what would you do? You'd told a bus conductor you'd run away from home, hoping he'd let you off the fare, but he just clucked and said, "Love, everyone in London's run away. What's so special about that?"

Down to your last few pounds, you'd splurged on a clairvoyant. Some girls at work had talked him up, touting his predictions as gospel. At first, you'd listened half-heartedly but when one woman came in sporting a diamond ring, just like the one the man had said she'd be given, your ears perked up. Maybe he would have access to the angels or the Face that seemed to have abandoned you years ago. Or even old Jamesie, wouldn't that be grand? Maybe he'd offer some inkling of hope for the future.

So after you'd finished the late shift, you walked the half mile to the alley where his office was. You found him inside, sitting in a dark room behind a table. His shaggy hair and crumpled clothes didn't fill you with much confidence but you put your money on the peeling wood and sat down. He'd better be good.

The clairvoyant, Mr. Mankiewicz, he was called, instantly stood up and starting pacing back and forth across the room. He seemed nervous, on edge, as he scratched the back of his scalp. Your heart beating hard in your chest, watching him.

"Headaches," he said. "Do you get headaches?"

You shook your head.

"I feel deep pain in the skull. You need a lot of protection."

Your palms felt clammy. "From what?" You tried but he'd already launched into a monologue.

"Do you have trouble remembering things?" He didn't wait for an answer. "I see your past, it's in a graveyard, buried under rubble. And your head…." He kept slouching from one wall to the other. "Light, yes light, it's streaming from your heart. But first, you have to walk through many doors, thick, heavy doors, one after another. You'll pass through them but it won't be easy or simple."

Doors? Your mind was scrambling, trying to make sense of his words. You wished he'd sit down, calm himself. "Oh!" He seemed to be on another tack now. "There you are!" Though he wasn't looking at you. "On top of a mountain…"

Now you were convinced he was a fraud. You'd never been drawn to mountains. If he'd said rivers, lakes, anything to do with water, you might have believed him.

"Yes, on a mountain top, arms stretched up and out… like Jesus. And light pouring off you…. But first, the long journey."

You were already standing when he finally glanced at you, as if the sight of your shaking body was almost too much for him. "Get protection!" He'd yelled after you as you slammed the door.

A waste of hard earned dosh, you told yourself, but still your heart wouldn't slow down. You had to get out of this strange city.

Yet another place you didn't belong. Grateful for the street lamps guiding your way, you found yourself opening the door of a phone box and your fingers, as if in a trance, dialing home.

A hullabaloo on the other end. Your mother spewing concern, then anger, recrimination, and finally relief that she knew your whereabouts.

She put Da on the line and something in his voice broke the steel wall of your heart. Your face wet, sniffling, you tried to explain.

"We know, Eily, we know," Da cut in, "we saw it in the Post. Young woman's car slams into farmer's sheep."

"But how did you know it was me?"

"Ah, we'd a letter from Old Maher last year, telling us you were well and safe. It was in the news. Once we got word of old Maher's passing, sure we put two and two together."

"Really?" You inhaled in surprise.

"Yeah, we found the farmer. No one was sure if the brakes had given up or the accelerator'd been broken. And we don't need to know. Anyway, Mr. Callaghan was raging."

"God! What'd he say?"

"A half dozen sheep injured – not badly – and one dead."

You could hardly imagine how you did that, much less how you were responsible for it.

"Anyway, after a lot of blarney, we took care of it for you, girl."

You learned later that the farmer was an admirer of your father's rugby prowess on the field. Still, he was out six sheep, and one permanently. He wanted compensation. So Da, you heard, cycled into town, drew out the bulk of his retirement fund and had a bank draft made out to Mr. Callaghan.

You were a puddle of tears and remorse, your throat cracking with the news. Inside you, something melted and something else died.

Da had wangled your address out of you and truth be told, it was a fine surprise when you saw the envelope with his handwriting on it in the staff room.

Mo Chailín Bán,
You've been gone from us a long time now. You should consider coming home. Whatever may have passed between us, you're always welcome at our hearth.
As I said, we tracked down Farmer Callaghan after reading about his loss in the paper. I went myself to the Bank of Ireland and paid him what he was out for his sheep. So you're all squared away, girl. Jesus tells us forgiveness is our greatest weapon in this world so let's put the past where it belongs – behind us. It's time to move forward, Eily. Bring yourself home soon, why don't you?

You'd gone back to the blueblack air of Dublin, deep scars tarred over with practice. Waiting at the doorstep your father was, and he took one look at you, scrawny, disheveled, and started weeping. "Mother," he whispered, his arms nearly crushing you, "feed the girl a steak."

You knew you'd won the jackpot then. All the while growing up, Liam got the steak being the boy, while you were dished up liver and onions every time.

He hefted a couple of your bags into his arms and said, "Don't worry, girl. We'll do it like the university people."

"How's that, Da?"

"By degrees."

There was a rug draped over the red doorstep, you still remember the pattern, a faded rectangle with tigers on it. They had puce, fiery tongues that stuck out. "We've rolled out the red carpet for you, so we have." And inside you went like royalty, only to find a cake with thirty-one candles on it, one for each month you'd been away. Da's idea. He was a good man, still is.

Sure, you'd had a happy childhood, hadn't you? Food usually on the table at mealtimes. Liam cracking stupid jokes over supper, even if they were a bit colorful. Ma in her apron racing round the kitchen like a hasty chicken. What had possessed you to ditch it all? Was it because you'd been failing exams at school, some sort of shame? You couldn't quite remember. When you tried to conjure the past, all you found was mud. Well, you'd missed the Leaving Cert so you'd not have a hope in hell of going to university any more. What darkness lurked in you that you always seemed to invite trouble, even if you weren't looking for it?

And then you met Rory. He ran the marketing department at the new high tech company on the south side, where you'd gotten work as a telephonist. He was shorter than you, with a scraggly blond beard and piercing eyes. He wore that air of confidence that seemed exclusive to Americans and when he insisted you join him for lunch one day, you dropped everything and went. You enjoyed driving round the city in his Triumph Spitfire, and he filling your head with stories of life in Oregon. You drank in his every word, mesmerized.

One day, he dangled the one carrot that still seemed tasty. "Anyone can go to college there, easy as pie," he said, as if he was talking about boiling a kettle.

"Even if you never finished secondary school?" You'd been longing to put your mind to use again. For a while now, it had been a cloudy swamp, floating on visions of howling sheep and little else.

You'd been so bored answering telephones with the stale glut of recited words that you'd started to mess around. When a man with a south side accent asked for the managing director, you'd told him he was out. "Do you know when he'll be *bach?*" He'd said in his upper crust accent and you couldn't help yourself, it sounded so much like the composer, you'd replied, "I'm not sure. He's not very musical!"

"Even without high school." Rory had laughed. "You just take a test – the SATs – and you're in."

The notion of going to university there – when all roads in Ireland were closed to you – rummaged around in your head for weeks. Rory said there were scholarships and financial aid available too.

So when he invited you to go with him when he returned to Oregon, you thought long and hard about it. You'd never belonged here, never fit in. And yet there was a kind of rough-hewn loyalty to family. They had their failings, granted, but hadn't they been good to you, bailing you out after you'd mown down those innocent animals? Hadn't Da spent his last few pennies on you? Didn't Ma dish you up extra helpings of dessert every so often?

Once Da had even cycled in the pouring rain with you to Whitehall so you could catch the nearest bus to the airport swimming pool and he'd taken your bike after you boarded and wheeled it all the way home for you. It warmed your heart to re-conjure such kindness.

And yet. Rory eventually wore you down with his tales of prosperity, opportunity, the chance to explore a fresh life, maybe to put the past behind you once and for all, to begin again.

That short holiday in Oregon stretched into years at university, earning credit for, imagine this, tennis and skiing. And libraries of books to ingest. The scholarship fund's one condition was that you tour community centers and speak about Irish Life and Culture. You enjoyed the elderly folks, who tried to fix you up with their sons and teased you over your accent. You were surprised they didn't consider they had one too.

The question most often asked was had you seen a leprauchán. You loved to tell them of that great answer a country woman gave in the early 1920's. When she was asked by a folklorist if she believed in fairies, she shot back, "I do not!" And after a pause, "but sure, they exist anyway."

You didn't have time for fairies any more. America took you in like a new love, tentatively, even if you had a bit of a time understanding each other at first. The first day in Journalism 101, the teacher said, "You're not in Ireland now. Use American spelling." It took a while to remember to drop the 'u' in color and humor but you savored the economy of language here. How everything was abbreviated, efficient. Light became Lite. It saved time, energy. You got the hang of it and swilled the wondrous word Wow! around on your tongue like sugar. Even with two languages to choose from, there wasn't a whiff on an expression to equal such wonder back home.

You'd finally realized your childhood dream, arrived in the land of transformation. You could be whoever you fancied here. The past was rapidly becoming like tea that had steeped too long – cloudy, sour. Here was your chance to imagine a new script for the tapestry of days to unravel. The little boy you'd babysat for a while couldn't pronounce your name so you changed it, just like that. One minute, you were breathing through the habit of Eily, short, precise, clipped. The next, you'd slipped into the meandering garment of Ella, gentle hills rising and dipping and rising again.

When someone would ask your name, Ella would slip off your tongue like velvet. It sounded more adult, sophisticated even. But when asked about growing up in Ireland – people seemed enchanted by the old country – you'd trouble dredging up more than a handful of memories. And always the same ones: Kiara's family's Volkswagen 2609Z; the sheer satin of your Communion panties; and of course, Banjo, the love of your life. But for some reason, you couldn't even conjure his face any more. It had blurred into the mist of dead memory.

One scholarship led to another. After years of not reading beyond front page news, you rediscovered your love of books. They were bountiful and new, not like the shelves of Drumcondra

Library with worn out covers and pages missing. You tried for a while to study elementary education. You'd always loved children, their uncalculated ways, but the practicums in schools were disappointing. You couldn't keep the boys' and girls' names straight. There were so many divided families. And they were always telling you they were a quarter one nationality and three quarters another.

You were glad to have just the one country. It took ages to realize that you too were a hybrid. If you ever wrote a book about your parents, it'd have to be called The Anglo-Irish Treaty. It had charmed you over the years watching them joke around and have a laugh together, she washing dishes, he on his stool, carefully drying them. They'd found a way to make peace from their differences.

You came back to your first love – poetry. Da used to be always quoting lines from the rich store he'd had to memorize in school. He was mad about the Romantics, Wordsworth's nature odes, Shelley's deep meditations, and he knew most poems by heart. Along he'd trot in his measured tones, Keats' reaming off him like water, *My heart aches, and a drowsy numbness pains my sense.* He always had a yen for the darker elements, it seemed, but it surprised you that he and Liam shared a love of the same poem. For some reason – you couldn't say why, it had been a long while – there was bitter blood between them. The line they pegged out of that laborious Elegy On A Country Churchyard, by Gray, was a morbid one, *Full many a flower was born to blush unseen and waste its sweetness on the desert air.* And somehow, it spoke to you too, imagining a tiny crocus blasted by high winds, graciously yielding itself. Alone, unnoticed, never to be appreciated by anyone.

Ah sure, those days were long gone. Liam became a doctor, he was always one for the learning, and he took off for the United Arab Emirates to earn his fortune. Last time you saw him, he said he was no spring chicken and if he was to get a woman, he'd need hard cash. You'd offered to help him find one. In fact, you'd spent quite a bit of time vetting his potential wives. When he was flush, he'd take the three of you out to a slap up meal, sometimes at

Locks on the canal. You'd drink red wine and end with port and a platter of cheeses. You'd chat about poetry and plays and sometimes politics.

And afterwards, you'd hop on the back of Liam's Goldwing and wave to the poor girl left standing on the street. Only you never agreed on the same woman. To be honest, you were a little bit in love with him yourself. He had eyes that seemed almost Asian, thin almond colored slits. And the contours of his face, honed, defined, well, they bespoke an elegance far removed from Ireland. You'd told him once you'd be his wife if he hadn't been a brother but he just brushed you off, saying, "G'way outta that, ye hussy!" In the end, you were just grateful to spend time with him.

Once he became smitten with Ann Kirkland from the avenue. She had a blue eye and a brown eye and braided hair she wore like a tail down her back. But she'd been into someone else. Liam had locked himself in his room, playing LPs so loud the O'Reilly's complained. Your own heart twinged, watching him, struggling between wanting to convince the girl she was making a big mistake, and a faint sadness she wasn't you.

Poor bloke came to a grim crossing, though, on his lonely road. It was back when there were all those AIDS scares. Being a doctor exposed to all kinds of viruses, he'd taken a test and it came back positive. God, he was in such a white heat that time, he nearly faded away. If it wasn't for the Guinness, he'd have been a goner. Like its name, it kept him stout. And he'd been seeing this girl from Gorey. Breda. She worked as a hotel receptionist. She thought she might have the dread disease too, being as they'd been intimate. They were a right pair. He took her to Paris and on the Champs Elysées, she said, "Liam, sure, if we're both going to die, we might as well go down together." He was touched by that so he proposed to her there and then.

They got married but you were already in America and missed the wedding. Turned out neither of them was sick and even though they were like chalk and cheese, sure, the damage was done.

Rory was fascinating, different, exciting but you were not in love. Who knows if you were capable of real love in those years? Men were a foreign species. You squashed down your breasts with a tight vest and always wore the same baggy sweater, no matter how many colorful dresses Rory had his secretary choose for you. And making love, well, that was unthinkable. You hewed to Da's dictates back then, save yourself for the one you'll marry. Oh, the idealist you were. And Rory was pleased he'd found himself a virgin.

For Christmas, he took you to a cabin on Mount Hood. The river sang as it flowed past the porch. Fir trees were bundled in snowy robes. You snuggled by the blazing fire, sipping on hot toddys. On Christmas Day, Rory presented you with a pair of baby's booties instead of the usual ring, a hint – or a hope – of things to come. You weren't sure you loved him enough and besides he was Jewish. What would your father say? There was no way you could get hitched without his seal of approval. You hesitated, said you needed time to think.

You wrote a long letter to Da, asking his advice. The only area you'd be guaranteed firm counsel from him was in matters of religion.

An envelope with Da's handwriting arrived by return post.

Eileen,

I have received your surprising news of January 8. I'm sorry to say that I am not equipped to advise you on the marriage of a Catholic to a Jew. The best I can offer – and this is vital, girl – is to ask either Father Talbot over here or find a parish priest in Oregon. Sit him down and get all the ins and outs before you make such an irrevocable decision.

Please let me know how you proceed.

All my love,

But you never got the chance to hunt down a liberal priest. In the new year, Rory had business in Dublin and went – without you – to visit the folks. Liam cornered him within the first hour, told him to kick you out, that you'd never marry him.

Back in Portland, Rory slept in a separate bedroom and his periodic advances met with rejection. But after months living, breathing, eating in the same house, he wore you down. You couldn't deny you liked the feel of his fingers tracing shapes along your back or the taste of his tongue angling round yours. Eventually one sunny afternoon in the loft, you lay down together and he wormed his way inside. It felt strange and yet familiar, the heft of his body flat against yours, the squirming and sighing. He said he'd know when to remove himself and in the heat of the long build-up, you finally yielded.

But the fireworks of sensation that flooded every cell of your being convinced you that you had conceived a child. Rory laughed and brushed it off. Weeks later, when you began to feel sick in the mornings, you had a test. It came back positive.

At first you were elated. You'd always wanted to be a mother. And if Rory wasn't the man of your dreams, then it was fate and you'd been willing to surrender to it. You quit smoking, read every book you could find on how to have a healthy pregnancy. Your life was being laid out before you, not in the way you'd imagined, but who were you to deny destiny?

Only Rory didn't see it that way, not at all. He reminded you that you'd been hesitant to marry him and now, he said, you were feeling trapped and doing it for all the wrong reasons. He nudged you towards terminating the pregnancy. When you refused, he carted you off to see a counselor. This woman insisted that you have extensive therapy if you did not keep the child. Given your strict Catholic background, she said, it could wreak havoc with your emotional and mental stability.

What with the hormonal shifts erupting inside, you were a walking time bomb, crying at every little thing. You remember driving back to Rory's house, feeling like the bottom had dropped out of the world. That cliff at the hill's crest started to look inviting. What would Da say? It would ruin him, the shame of his only daughter having a baby out of wedlock. And you'd no money to go home anyway. And what about your studies, which were so precious to you? Your mind had been expanding but your womb was gaining ground. Rory promised to find the best therapist in town if you had an abortion. With no resources to have the child alone, in a foreign country, you saw no way out.

So, heartbroken, you read everything you could find on the formation of the fetus. At six weeks, there was barely an embryo forming. If you were to do it, it would have to be soon.

In between periods of vomiting and arguing with Rory, you made an appointment at the abortion clinic. That Saturday morning remains seared in your brain, the heavy clouds hovering like Da's black moods, the scent of rain in the air. The counselor had advised you to be the last one seen so there'd be fewer people around and Rory accompany you. When you parked the car and walked towards the entrance, you met a group of men and women bearing signs of dead babies, and hefting huge signs, *Abortion Is A Sin. Repent Now Before You Go To Hell. Don't Be A Murderer.*

They closed in, a pack of glowering wolves, and you could imagine your own father there in the midst of them, bearing his own placard promising damnation for what you were about to do. The notion almost broke you. Sick and shivering, you let Rory push the crowd off you as you beat a path to the door.

The procedure itself was ridiculous. A man in a white coat vacuuming or something and then shouting, "I can't find anything. It's too early. There's nothing in there."

Afterwards, a kindly nurse offered a supply of contraceptives. You flung them across the room. "If you think I'm ever going to make love again, you've another think coming!" But emotionally charged vows, however sincere in the moment, rarely last.

And then home again, if you could call it home. The bathroom toilet drinking up all your vomit. And a call from the clinic. They forgot to do a D&C, they said, to vacuum out the remains. You had to go back again. Now.

You could barely stand up. Rory handed you your coat as the phone rang again. This time, out of the blue, it was Ma, ringing from Dublin. "I just felt like seeing how you are, Eileen." That was the final straw. The timing of it. Back then, phone calls were rare, saved for Christmas and birthdays. She had a psychic streak, your mother. Something in her knew though you didn't dare tell her. She adored Rory, flirting with him when he'd visited Dublin, you heard, as if she were still a chaste schoolgirl. You just wept into the speaker and said you couldn't talk for long, you had somewhere to go.

Months later, when you were working across town, selling pens or some such thing, you were on the phone, reaming off the benefits of purchasing whatever it was when you felt something erupt inside and ooze out between your legs. Your pants were soaked. You pulled your skirts in close and stumbled towards the bathroom. Blood, great big clots of it, were falling between your thighs, a waterfall of crimson.

You'd called Rory in a panic but his secretary said he was in an important meeting and couldn't be disturbed.

So you took two buses home, leaving a trail of blood in your wake.

You never did see the counselor. Rory changed his mind about therapy in the end. Though after you'd moved out, it was inevitable, he suggested you continue making love.

At some point, you found a part time job at The Oregonian newspaper, in advertising. The work was mundane but the small group of you who wrote copy got along well. George was a sweet man from Alaska, the most exotic place you could imagine back then. He brought you little gifts – a box of pastilles, crayons

— and left funny notes on your desk. It took you a while to realize he liked you. You'd catch a bus out to Hawthorne on Wednesdays to do laundry and always share a good laugh. He was humorous in a childish kind of way. He was always asking you about your past.

"You must've been adorable as a girl," he'd say and you'd wince. An image of you, young, scrawny, looking disconsolately at your reflection in the glass and wishing mirrors had never been invented. But George was so charming, you'd ply him with the few cheery tales you had at your disposal. You half thought about going out with him but then you met Spencer.

Spencer was in your poetry class at Portland State. And god, could he write. He had a brilliant mind and vivid blue eyes that glared from behind his round-rimmed glasses. He wrote about exotic places in Mexico, where he'd traveled, and you struggled to keep up with his wild metaphors. An arrow lunged into your chest as he talked. You were smitten. You'd meet on Friday nights at Produce Row. Pitchers of beer would drown away all shyness. You had to drink milk beforehand to keep up with him.

You'd stagger back to your place, laughing, he full of lectures on existentialism and Nietchze's Superman. You were bowled over by his intellect. He wrote beautiful, spare lines about Lake Patzcuaro and San Miguel de Allende, places he'd hitchhiked to as a teenager. He informed you he intended to write the Great American Novel. You truly believed he would.

One afternoon, he arrived at your door, all flush-cheeked, and said he'd submitted poems for The Academy of American Poets Award. Great, you said. "Wish I'd known about it. I could have entered that Irish sequence I wrote." You'd been working on a series of persona poems, poking fun at the Irish stereotypes.

The deadline for submission was that afternoon. Spencer had emptied a bottle of Chardonnay into two glasses by then and you were half-sozzled. "Sure, why don't I give it a try too?" The grand prize was $100 plus a ceremony, where the awards would be delivered by a famous writer you both admired.

So you plucked the poems out of the cabinet, dizzily typed your name on the cover sheet, and you slouched arm in arm up to the English department and slid the envelope under the door, Spencer riffing different acceptance speeches, some witty, some biting, as you went. You remember laughing as you skipped all the way home.

Weeks passed with no response. So long that you'd forgotten all about it.

Eventually you and Spencer moved into a small upstairs apartment on Columbia Street. He wasn't working so you paid most of the bills. You'd go out drinking and talk about having children. He'd get all morose after a few, the way you remembered Irish men in the pubs at home. One night, he leered, "If we ever split, I'd fight you in court every step of the way to keep the kids."

You said nothing, let him ramble on, knowing deep down there was a warning here but what could you do? You were in love.

And then the phone call. Spencer was out when Professor Gilliam – a robust, serious man – rang.

"Prepare yourself, young lady." He said sternly.

"For what?"

"The judges were unanimous. Your Irish Sequence won The Academy's highest prize for students."

"You're joking me!" You fell back against the cabinet.

"Indeed I'm not. Everyone was captivated by the characters you portrayed – so vital and lifelike."

"Janey Mac!" was all you could muster.

"Well, aren't you delighted, young miss?"

"I suppose so…" but in your mind, you were already trying to figure out how to break the news to Spencer, who had loftier dreams of literary success than you.

"And if I'm not mistaken," Gilliam droned on, "your, ahem, boyfriend is the runner up."

Your heart sank. That made it all the harder. Who wants to be a runner up? Spencer just did not fit the bill.

"Em," you stalled, your mind spinning, "I don't suppose you'd be able to reverse the results?"

You were the wage earner for one thing. Having more money and a poetry win over Spencer would not go down well, you could feel it. He had a fierce pride. Your heart was pedaling a mile a minute.

Gilliam gave the heartiest laugh you'd ever heard from him. "Now it's you who's joking, isn't it?"

You tried to convince him you were serious but no amount of pleading would budge him. "The decision is final." So that was that.

Spencer was shocked, then surprised, but after a few drinks, he eased up, even offered a weak congrats, and began rehearsing his acceptance speech again. He wanted to impress that famous writer.

Not long after, George got wind of your thing with Spencer and he made a bold move. He'd heard you talk at length about how you'd love to live in San Francisco. He'd been there and was full of stories about the hills and the trams and the sunny weather. The state university had a Masters program in Poetry and you'd considered applying. One day, George arrived at work and said, "Guess what? I found a place in the Bay Area. I'm moving there."

Maybe he thought you would follow him, that your love of a place you'd never seen would lure you there, a ready made home. You did go down and see him once and made love in his little tower room. It was more powerful than you imagined possible. You told a friend in surprise and she said, "When someone loves you that much, you feel it."

Spencer and you continued the weekend drinking sprees. With him unemployed and prices rising, your meagre savings fizzled to a pittance. Most of it went to the liquor store on Broadway and it wasn't you doing all the boozing, Irish though you were.

Eventually it became clear there was only one door left to open and it read Exit. You came home from work one autumn evening

– you still remember the chill in the air – and told him you were leaving. He took it surprisingly calmly, said something vague but understanding. You offered to buy Chinese for supper. He nodded and off you went to Lao's.

You were gone for perhaps twenty minutes, half an hour at most. When you opened the front door, some animal instinct told you something was terribly wrong. Up the staircase, magazines and books were splayed open, pages ripped out. A library in tatters. You crept around the mess and stumbled upstairs.

And oh, the sight of what greeted you took your breath away. Chairs, table upturned, lamps on their sides, bulbs shattered, the vase of lilies you'd bought just the day before was a jigsaw of glass, stems flung about the room, cinnamon pollen smudged into the carpet.

You clambered over the wild mess and ventured into the bedroom where you found the wardrobe doors wide open, dresser drawers smashed against the mirror. Clothes in shreds on the mattress. No sheets or comforter in sight.

No Spencer either. You yelled who knows what. Shock does its unique number on people. The heft of pressure on your chest made it difficult to breathe. You kept moving, carefully, as if in a trance, the Chinese food cartons clutched to your ribs. Was this a terrible dream you'd wake from any minute? But wherever you cast your gaze, you found ruin.

Finally, in the bathroom, hunched over the toilet seat, a bottle of Seagrams glued to his lips, sat Spencer. His glasses – such charming round James Joyce spectacles, gold-rimmed – were askew on his nose. His face was scarlet. He wouldn't look at you.

You opened your mouth, taking in the ripped bath towel and the stink of piss, and nothing came out. How long you stood there before the retching in your throat made you vomit, you'll never know. Minutes maybe. Hours.

You put the food in the sink, turned around, and somehow floated back downstairs and out that door into the rest of your natural life.

You were fortunate to find a room in a house on the other side of town. The tiny square window looked out on a lovely garden next door and you imagined all the flowers dormant in the winter earth, just biding their time until they could blossom into their fullness.

Several months passed and it seemed like things were settling down again. You kept busy, with classes and writing and work at the paper. But Spencer knew your schedule well. You started to see him lurking in the shadows when you'd leave the swimming pool. Some days, he'd follow as you walked, always a few feet behind. It was unnerving, as if he wanted to make sure you'd never forget him. And then the dozens of bleeps on the phone machine, but they were all hang ups. You knew it was him. He was starting to haunt you.

Still it was a shock one evening to find him leaning against your car when you left the office. You had no desire to talk to him and slid through the driver's door and turned on the ignition quickly. But as you pulled out from the curb, Spencer lunged onto the hood and leered through the window. There you were driving down 23rd Avenue with a monster on your car, his eyes crazed and you screaming at him to *get off now for God's sake!* You couldn't even see where you were going.

You screeched to a halt in the middle of the road, praying the cars behind would yield. Though it had only been a matter of minutes, it felt like an eternity. Spencer had been shouting wildly through the glass the entire time. You were in such shock that you barely remember what happened. Only a shuffle of bodies, men pulling Spencer off the hood and dragging him out of the road and he yelling threats at you the entire time.

Somehow you found your way home, shaking, all ragged breath, and fell into a chair. Next day, you went to the courthouse and had a restraining order issued. That helped for a while but those things expire. Spencer still called but you never picked up. You wondered what it was in you that could have attracted

– or been attracted to – such a maniac. But no answers surfaced.

You were still convinced that he bordered on genius but the delicacy of his mental state raised major issues. For years afterwards, he would find you, wherever you moved to, even to other towns. The phone would ring and with a sinking feeling, you'd hear his voice on the other end, "Guess who?"

Professor Gilliam suggested graduate school. He pointed you to colleges that offered fellowships so you'd be funded and still be legal.

So you applied to a variety of schools and ultimately chose Johns Hopkins because, you hesitate to admit, they offered a teaching assistantship you could live on. You packed a few belongings, gave the rest away, and flew across the country to Baltimore.

A year later, M.A. in hand, you skipped graduation. With your teaching assistant's savings, you bartered for a battered Volkswagen beetle. The front bumper was dented and it exhaled a charm of fumes when you drove. But it did drive and it brought back fond memories of Kiara's family car back in Dublin, though that was a Rolls Royce by comparison. With nowhere else to go, you'd packed up your poetry books and hightailed it back to Oregon.

Bright as you were in some subjects, you weren't doctorate material and you knew it. But without a student visa, you couldn't stay in America. A dizzying swarm of men kindly offered to marry you but you were keen to hold out for the Right One. Who could live up to the charm of Da, with his boyish humor and poetic soul? Occasionally, Cupid's arrow pierced you bullseye in the chest and you'd been bonkers over this bloke or that but it didn't last. You always packed your bags once the talk of you know what came up. Maybe it was because you couldn't imagine waking up on the same pillow for a lifetime with any of them. Or maybe it just meant none of them was your father.

After using up the twelve months allotted to apply your degree, you were running out of options. Maybe it was time to give up on living in America. You looked into airfares home. They were not cheap so you decided to wait. But the days wore on and with one week left on your visa, you got woken in the night by the telephone. It was Ma in Dublin, holding a letter, she said, from the American Embassy. You had won a permanent visa in a lottery. Who could explain such a miracle? Maybe best to put it down to the luck of the Irish.

Being a fatalist, you'd been prepared to go back to the doom of Dublin but no, the universe had other plans. So you bought a bottle of good Cabernet and settled into a small apartment in the northwest.

You began teaching at the Community College, Freshman Composition. But eventually you worked your way up to Creative Writing and Poetry. You enjoyed the students, often middle-aged men and women who worked full time and wanted to better themselves. You'd have a laugh most days, especially at your VW. It had a bumper sticker that read, *If you're Prince Charming, knock on the window and kiss me.* You'd tried to pry it off without success. One cheeky student always signed his papers as P.C. You let him know he wasn't.

One facet of American living that beguiled you was the endless coffee refills. You'd never liked it much in Ireland but it was robust here, especially if you drank it black: it filled out all those empty spaces inside. And oh, those buffets. All you could eat. A waitress once asked as you were leaving Izzi's, "Are you stuffed yet?" Little did she know you lived to stuff yourself. Somewhere along the way, food had become a constant lover, always poised to seduce. And you succumbed over and over but alas, there was no afterglow.

People swore they remembered you by the particular food that obsessed you. For a while, it was cheese, any cheese, and carrots.

Nothing else but water. Then you graduated to salad bars. You'd eat almost nothing from Monday to Thursday and come Friday, you'd head over to The Jazz Quarry and almost empty their supplies. It took your stomach the whole weekend to recover. Feast or famine, that was you. In graduate school, apples were the fruit of your eye. You bought them by the bushel at Safeway and chewed till your teeth hurt. That was the year nothing but Eve's hand-me-downs from Eden crossed your tongue. At least meat was off the menu. You hadn't been able to stomach a shred of animal flesh ever since those gored sheep insinuated themselves into your dreams.

Maybe it was the loneliness of this new country. Maybe it was habit, keeping your mouth occupied. It kept you from saying things, admitting things you might regret. It's amazing you didn't swell up like a Michelin woman. It became almost an act of strength, to see how much you could ingest.

It took many years of food extravaganzas for you to end up in Overeaters Anonymous. You had a roommate who was a regular in A.A. She would find you in the kitchen at all hours, poring over spicy tofu or ice cream. Once after a marathon chocolate session, you'd said half-joking, "Do you think I have a problem with eating?"

Katherine was an artist. She used to leave notes for you in the morning with witty illustrations. She took a pencil from the drawer and drew a straight line. "One end," she said, "indicates No Problem. The other, a very big problem. You," she dug the pencil point into the paper, "are here." You gazed at the gray dot that sealed your fate. It was hovering midway between the mid point and Big Problem. To be honest, you were shocked. You'd expected her to flick off the question with a laugh. You sat staring at the page, your stomach making strange, hissing sounds.

You learned later that denial is a big part of the addict's arsenal. And the overeater's. Denying all those feelings that were too excruciating to bear. Food pads the discomfort with a coating somewhat like potato mash.

So you snuck into an Overeaters Anonymous meeting, covering your face with a hood. You didn't want to be identified and thus, labeled. Shame is no understudy in an eater's play.

The speaker gave a detailed history of how her chronic obsession with food had ruined her life. You listened intently. She cornered you after the meeting (it's protocol to welcome newcomers) and swished in your ear, "3 – 0. Three meals a day, nothing in between. Just ask God for help."

You'd had about six already and it was only early evening. You skulked home, convinced you couldn't make it till breakfast without a bite of something passing your lips. But somehow evening melted into night into morning and by some miraculous grace, not a morsel passed your lips. A force greater than you must have been helping, you reasoned, knowing you could never have done that by sheer force of will.

And so you found yourself at O.A. meetings regularly. You were a varied bunch but you all had one thing in common – a dis-ease, as it was called. So you dropped your separate selves and surrendered, prayed, shared stories. Slowly, it became a habit, a good habit. You found a sponsor to call when temptation raised its voice. You had a phone list of names. Eaters tend to isolate, you learned, and so reaching out was difficult but once you got in a groove, you found it helped to chat with someone who was enduring similar seductions to yours.

After meetings, people would often ask you to share more about Ireland. Somehow the country glittered with a million myths that everyone seemed eager to unearth. You'd share the happiest times you could re-conjure – the surprise trip to the sea on the back shelf of Kiara's family car; Banjo, your first and deepest love; swinging in the carnival boats at Portmarnock the day your mother dropped everything to take you and Liam in a taxi to the sea.

But after you got home, you'd spend hours lying on your bed, unable to dredge up a single experience when you were four, five, six. Of course, you remembered Banjo, your true love. But try as you might, not a single image of him could you dredge up. He'd become a phantom. And those satin panties you adored wearing on your Communion, you could still feel their smooth texture but the day itself had become a blur. Eight, nine, ten. What happened to that young girl, you wondered, the lost years trailing out behind you, a blank canvas.

It almost hurt to scour those years, struggling to locate a key that would unlock the story of your past. It was buried somewhere and you were convinced if you tried hard enough, the secret opening would reveal itself.

One night, you jolted out of a vivid dream. It had something to do with the lilacs in your back garden who kept you company all those years ago. They were swaying in a soft dance, fluid as water, and vague as an Impressionist painting.

Next day, you used your meager savings to call home. "Mum," you began. "Do you remember the woman I used to chat with in the lilac bush?"

An embarrassingly long pause during which you could hear her breathing and almost watch the machinery of her mind as she calculated the best response.

"What was her name? For the life of me, I can't recall it."

Silence.

"Mum?"

"Eileen," she said in the softest tone I'd heard from her. "Eileen, that... was just... *fan*tasy."

Oh your poor, dear mother, thinking you were off your rocker, still believing in fairies and the like.

You had to laugh. "It's okay, Ma..."

"Mum!" She never lost a chance to set you straight.

"I was just thinking of how kind she was to me. She was there when I needed her."

"It's Mrs. Mulligan you're talking about, isn't it? Well, you don't need her now, do you?"

No, but you could have used a loving mother. Instead, you shrugged your shoulders, sighed, and said goodbye.

Eventually you grew weary poring down the tunnel of your past and put it down to poor memory, letting yourself cherish the few dusty windows you could still open. Maybe the mind is selective: it focuses solely on the positive, and surely that was a good thing. Your sponsor commented once that you spoke about your father a lot but rarely mentioned Ma. She wondered if your mother was dead.

And then the invitation arrived.

Mo Chailín Eily,
 cén chaoí bhfuil tú? We're all well here. Mother is off in England but I'm keeping the home fires burning, a few spuds in the pot, the kettle on the boil. It's a soft day here, drizzling on and off. The last of the summer flowers have died off. It's not quite a 'season of mists and mellow fruitfulness,' but sure, we're glad for whatever's offered. Isn't that right?

 Eileen, I wanted to see about Christmas. It's ages since you've graced our front door, girl. I just had an insurance policy mature. I'm thinking it'd go a long way towards bringing you home for the holidays.

 I can safely say your mother and Liam would be as happy to see you, child, as I would myself.

 Have a think on it.

All my love,

It had been years since you'd set foot in Ireland and a quiet longing planted itself in your heart. For hours, you'd imagined the four of you, Mum, Da, Liam and yourself, in the sitting room by the fire, pulling crackers and putting on party crowns. Da would pull out his annual cigar, making his juvenile jests. The tree would glisten with powdered snow, fairy lights winking as if they too were in on the joke. There were still some shaped like bells that Mum brought over from England after she married. They were weathered but you could read the little love words on them if you squinted.

You wrote back, thanking Da for his generosity. He'd always been kind, not just to you. He put half his paycheck into the donation plate after Mass. You don't know how he managed, really.

But Ma would have none of it. She rang, almost hysterical, saying, "you can't possibly come home. I've enough to consider what with the turkey and gravy and trimmings. There's no room for vegetarian food."

You'd make your own meals then. But no, she said, it was enough work, Lord knows, to manage everything already. She was not getting any younger. You would not be welcome at the table, and that was the end of all talk about it.

The news nearly sent you into an eating frenzy again. But you called your sponsor and sobbed for hours. She listened patiently. You spent the holidays, not where you wanted to but where you were wanted.

On rough days, Da's regular letters kept you going

My dearest Eily,

Thank you for your lovely letter of December 9. It's nice you can spend the holiday with friends. I'll be helping the new parish priest, Father Kennedy, to set up the altar for Christmas Day. And of course, yours truly will be the premier officiant at Communion!!!

We've had a spot of rough weather, big storms in the west. But as they say, if winter comes, can spring be far behind? One of these days the crocuses will pop their heads out and we'll know it's official!!!!

> *Child, the same moon that rises over Tom Kelly's chimney appears in your sky too. We're always looking at the same moon and can remember each other that way.*
>
> *With all my love,*

What moon? It hardly ever shone over there, the way the sky was always bruised with clouds. And what use was it even if two people put their attention on the same thing if they remained half a world apart?

Still, you relished his missives, the broad, expansive swirl of his letters on the page, the juvenile jokes, the usual news about upkeep of the old homestead, as he called it, and the parish goings on. He didn't gossip like a lot of the women in scarves, huddled in their rugby scrum, heads together, smoke from their cigarettes wisping skywards as they fed each other juicy tidbits.

His letters were long and often he'd throw in a line from a poem you both loved. *Hail to Thee, Blithe Spirit. Bird, thou never wert, that from Heaven or near it, pourest forth thy full heart, in profuse strains of unpremeditated art.* Still, there was a certain formality to his epistles, not quite business like — they were too friendly, too strewn with jokes for that — but it was as if he put on his Sunday shirt to write. For a farmer's son, he wrote eloquently and never misspelled a word. You had an eagle eye for that.

Your favorite part, every time, no matter how many letters you received that bore the same insignia, was his sign off, *With all my love, Daddy.*

All my love. As if he was handing over the heft of his heart, its light and shadowed shards, time and again, for you to cosset and keep. And oh, you did, scooping up the breakage in your willing arms, kissing the words as if they were 22 carat gold.

You couldn't say the same for your mother's missives. They arrived in her tiny, elegant handwriting but were sparse and lacking in affection. She didn't seem to lament your absence one bit. No matter how often you wrote to tell her you loved her, she never responded in kind. It was a mystery. You'd always craved her love – you know, the one who withholds is the one we most desire – and she'd always denied it.

Your father, on the other hand, shared his thoughts – if not his intimate feelings – in copious, overwritten displays, laden with exclamatives. You hung on every word, embracing the envelope his special hand had graced.

There was one man – infinitely older than you – whom you did move in with for a while. You had a notion to challenge yourself, to see if you could stay in a relationship for more than nine months. Steve was a skilled woodworker and though he was frugal, he kept a simple but attractive home. In winter, you used to keep the oven door open to heat the kitchen. Steve lived to travel and you shared many a lovely road trip, you reading stories to him as he drove, him helping you critique them as by then, you were a consulting editor for a literary journal.

You'd pull over by the side of a road and Steve would find a cosy nest – a field or a swath of tall grasses by some trees – and you'd make love, the vast heavens starring down on you. He built an Adironack canoe, which was curved in all the right places, elegant as a woman. He named it *Janey Mac,* a Dublin expression, kind of like Wow! that you used probably too often. His friends looked puzzled, wondering who Janey was and if Steve was having an affair. You both just laughed about it.

Sometimes he'd travel internationally and you'd stay home to write. He'd send postcards glutted with words, barely room for a stamp. They were newsy, informative, funny. It made your day to open the mailbox and find one, usually with a stunning picture on front. Vicarious travel, it was, and you loved it.

Your neighbor, Janet, had a literary escort business. It sounds racy but really, it required ferrying writers with new books around town, taking them to interviews, feeding them, sometimes doing their laundry. Janet hired you part time and you savored the chance to chat intimately with every writer you met. Some of them were heroes of yours. Strangely, though they proffered their phone number and implored you to send them your own writing, you never did.

One older man, who was renowned for his crime series, charmed your heart when you picked him up at the estimable Heathman Hotel. You were still driving the old VW station wagon and as this famous writer sat himself down in the passenger seat, the glove box plopped open and reams of papers, dental floss, and half eaten candy bars came toppling out onto his lap. Now this gentleman was a dapper dresser and you were mortified.

But instead of chiding you or making a snide remark, he guffawed loudly and said, "If you drove anything better, I'd think you were a Republican!"

Many lovely encounters ensued – children's writers, investigative journalists, Pulitzer winners. At one point, you had a collection of signed first editions.

Another well known and respected novelist arrived one beautiful autumn day. He'd written about Vietnam in heart rending, poetic prose, so delicately rendered that he had acquired a large following. He was charming, boyish, flirty, feigning a profound insecurity as a way to inveigle himself. He refused to entertain any interviews unless you sat in intimate proximity to him. This of course entailed sitting on his bed in the hotel room, the one place from which he would grant an audience.

After the press had left, you shared a hearty supper, during which he regaled you with tales from the wild, playing his vulnerable little boy routine to lure you more close. Oh, he was a charmer, no doubt, and you were profoundly attracted, not by his looks, but by his brilliance and wit. But you'd made an internal commitment to remain in a relationship for more than the usual few months. You wanted to test yourself, remain with Steve, see if you were actually capable of staying put.

So you turned down this writer's advances. As it happened, Steve was a fan of this man's books and attended the reading he gave at Powell's.

X begged you to have a drink with him after the reading, to 'calm' him. Journalists from the Oregonian were in the audience and one of them – a talented food writer – beseeched you to have a one-on-one with him, though it wasn't on the schedule.

So you suggested this woman come to the Heathman bar later that night. X had tried to lure you to his room again. "You're seeing someone, aren't you?"

You nodded.

"I knew it!" He almost spat. "I could tell by the way you walk that you're getting it!"

That was enough. You stood up and went to meet the journalist who was only too happy to take his arm and lead him upstairs. He scribbled his address and number on a book cover and said, "If you ever break up with this guy, *please* call me."

Not long after that, Steve took off on a trip to Vietnam. You remember missing him at first and then realizing it was time. No matter how you argued with yourself, some automatic program – the Ella Exit, perhaps – had clicked into place. You found an apartment to share in southeast and made a deposit.

When you picked up Steve at the airport, he waltzed off the plane in a sporty beret, all smiles. It hurts to re-conjure this now but at the time, you simply told him you were finished. Although you couldn't feel it then, you feel – deeply – now the blow he experienced as if it had been you who'd been gut socked.

Your new roommate commented on how little emotion you evinced in the aftermath. In your memory, you did shed tears. Not like your mother who couldn't bear to be seen as vulnerable in any way. She wouldn't cry at funerals but saved her sorrows for her late night pillow. But it wasn't until many years later that you realized your roommate was right. You had a steel padlock on the door of your heart that engendered grieving, or perhaps, any deep feeling.

The years that followed are a haze now. You took one trip to the Wallowa mountains for the winter, where you'd been offered the position of Writer In Residence. You were given a cabin by the river as a place to write and in return, taught writing workshops in the surrounding towns – grade and high school visits, adults in the local bookstore. You loved it and were welcomed warmly, a surprise, as you'd heard newcomers were kept at a distance.

You later understood it was because you weren't just a blow-in but were there temporarily to contribute to the community. A sharp-tongued farmer offered back-handed invitations to visit his sheep and you watched lambs being ushered into the world, poor things. But you stroked each new born gently, as if you could somehow make up for the brutality you'd once visited on their kind.

You frequented a cafe there, which was renowned for its donuts. A tough woman stood sentinel by her baked creations on Sunday mornings, when there was a queue down the street. And she dished them up to those of her choosing. If you didn't meet her approval, then tough luck, buddy. A rotund man shuffled in ahead of you one day and she took one look and said, "By the looks of you, you won't be needing any of these. Next please."

Profound kindness also reared its head. That winter was particularly snowy and cold. Your ancient VW with bad tires skidded all over and barely made it across the bridge to your cabin. You had to be towed out once, much to the amusement of the locals. You eventually asked the owner of a motel on the front end of the bridge if you could park there and walk home. He grudgingly agreed.

When the term was up, you brought a box of chocolates around to thank the man for letting you use a parking space.

He nodded and as you were walking out the door, he shouted, "Ya better have that front tire looked at before ya head out. It's flat."

You shook your head. "No, it's fine, really. I've been driving it all winter."

"Yeah," he shot back, "and I've been pumping it up every morning."

When you returned to Portland, you upped your attendance at O.A., clocking several meetings a week. You couldn't fall off the wagon after all that work, tempting as it was. You slogged through the steps, one by one, made calls for help even when it was the last thing you wanted to do.

Gradually, you began to feel strong, independent, and looked forward to your three daily meals. You swam and cycled. Kundalini yoga became part of the daily routine, early morning cold showers, stretches, evening meditations. The first time you took a class, you'd walked out into the night air, a radiant stillness shrouding your every move. All of the street lamps seemed to be haloed in gold. You were in love. The yoga sets were challenging but they kept you busy. The mantras quieted your mind. Slowly, you were finding some discarded part of yourself again, and relishing it.

Yogi Bhajan brought the Kundalini teachings to the west and though he was a distant figure, almost mythic, you thanked him every day in your heart. The yoga sets were clearing out old garbage, you could feel it. Stories swirled of how tough, even brutal he could be with people, smashing their egos unapologetically. Still, you remained loyal to him, grateful for how clear, even happy, you felt after each session.

Then one miraculous evening, you found yourself in the same room with him. He was staying with your yoga teacher, who lived nearby. He sat in a regal white chair in the middle of the living room, dozens of Sikhs on the floor in a half moon around him. You were the only non-Sikh present. He spent a few minutes, answering questions, harshly, you thought.

He pointed at you and said, "You think too much."

You sat silently until he invited you to come forward. Asking for your birthdate, he said, softly, "Whatever you put your mind to, you can achieve." Somehow in his powerful presence, there was no fear. You drank in the love that wafted through him. Someone told him you were a writer. He said, "Cupid is not stupid," and suggested you write about different kinds of love.

He even offered a hand of friendship, telling you he'd like to share the book he'd written on the Golden Temple in India.

You left in awe, never taking him up on his generous suggestion. Too intimidated, perhaps. But you realized, as you walked out into the sparkling night, that he had given you the greatest gift already: he had been a true father, supportive, loving, encouraging. Something you'd not known until that miraculous evening.

One of the gurus in the Kundalini lineage, Guru Ram Das, had promised that whatever wish you dreamed up on his birthday, would come true, guaranteed.

Each year on October 9, you'd wish for a new dress or more income, until finally you decided to go for the gold. You made a fervent wish for Self-Realization, not even knowing what that meant. It would be a long, hard road until you did.

Several unmemorable Christmases in Portland came and went. Meanwhile, you'd slogged through the first eight of the Twelve Steps. It was a reckoning, to be sure. You had to surrender to a greater power than your weak and willful self. You'd taken a 'searching and fearless moral inventory' of every time you'd hurt or resented another person and then, as required, shared it with someone, in this case, a woman you barely knew, who listened patiently.

The Irish years before Jamesie's death remained misty as autumn. Ghosts hovering but never close enough to make direct contact. Most of your carefully written confession involved relationships. And a recurring pattern of hasty departure.

It was a test, to be sure, revealing the murky crannies of your past to a stranger. But as you'd been promised, a certain lightness descended afterwards, as if a weight you'd been lugging for eons had been airlifted off your back.

Da, however, much as you adored him, still pulled on your heart. You weren't sure if his letters helped or made you miss him even more. What was that magnetic pull to him, when you'd barely spent any time together in your growing up years? The one time he'd taken you to a John Wayne movie – and you'd been so excited, the pair of you out on the town together – he'd snored his way through the entire feature. It was just another puzzle to add to the maze in your head.

Eily mo chroí,
I won't go into family news as Mother will bring you up to date soon and I'm busy with end of the year taxes.
But I wanted to share a poem I came across in The Golden Treasury of Poems. I know you have a head for the good line and this one is a beauty.

Oft In The Stilly Night

Ere slumber's chair has bound me,
Fond Memory brings the light
of other days around me:

The smiles, the tears
of boyhood's years,
the words of love then spoken:
the eyes that shone,
now dimm'd and gone
the cheerful hearts now broken!

The last stanza really got to you. Da had never been one for emotion and yet here, a secret vulnerability was leaking its way out and onto the page.

I feel like one
who treads alone
some banquet-hall deserted,

> *whose lights are fled*
> *whose garlands dead*
> *and all but he departed!*

You read the careful script, each word piercing some hidden place inside your tired heart, until tears dripped out your eyes and sleep took you away from buried sorrow.

Climbing the Twelve Step path was a constant exercise in surrender, sometimes easy, sometimes stalling over each successive hurdle. But you kept stumbling onwards.

And then Step Nine reared its head, beckoning you to make amends to everyone you may have hurt in the past. For you, this mostly involved tracking down a long list of old boyfriends and making a sincere apology. The prospect filled you with dread but by this time, O.A. was your strongest lifeline.

Somehow, once you'd made the intention to wrestle this monster, miracles occurred. You'd call an ex and arrange to meet wherever he chose. Once you got the first few lines out, it came easily – explaining the dread disease and how it had affected your ability to be present; admitting mistakes, apologizing for your behavior, and for leaving them in the lurch – basically, being responsible for cleaning up the scum on your side of the street.

Most were open and receptive, some shrugged, uneasy at your uncharacteristic display of deep feeling. Others said not to worry about it; they'd been culpable too. Some were surprised at this newfound openness. One said, "Buy me a few beers and we'll call it quits."

For you, it brought up a depth of emotion you hadn't even been aware of – splaying the cold truth before each man, undefended, you understood for the first time the havoc you had wrought in so many lives. This time, as you walked away, you felt small, humbled.

But there was one man you just could not track down – the one whose child you had almost borne – Rory. Twenty years on, you'd almost given up hope of finding him again. You knew he'd married but there was no listing in the phone book.

And then, as if to test your faith in miracles one more time, there he was, right in front of you, the last man on your list: standing up to get his luggage as the plane landed in Chicago. You were en route to Ireland, where you'd secured a plum gig, teaching summer classes at the university near your parents' house. But seeing Rory here, two decades on, at the very airport you'd both arrived in America together, was a shock and a marvel.

"Rorrreeee!" you yelled down the plane, fearful he'd get off first and you'd lose him again in the crowd. Everyone turned, including him, to look at the mad hatter screaming her head off. You looked directly at him and nodded. He raised an eyebrow as if he wasn't sure who you were. You moved out to the aisle and nudged forward towards him, he all the while with his eyes glued to you.

"Don't you know me?"

He shook his head and then a light bulb flashed. "Ella? It can't be!"

You nodded, beaming from ear to ear. Maybe this much-touted higher power really was helping out.

You went for a drink in the airport lounge and you apologized profusely for the ways you'd behaved two long decades ago. Though it was a difficult time, a huge transition for you in the new land, you'd often judged him, accused him of meanness, control. It wasn't pleasant to cast a cold eye back on the arrogance of youth.

He waved it off. "We were both immature, weren't we?"

He had three children now and traveled so much, he said they'd probably be taking your college classes before he saw them again. They lived in London and were content though his life was mostly work these days.

"You seem happy." He eyed you curiously, as if he couldn't

quite match the young woman he'd struggled to love long ago with the one before him now.

"I am, all the more for seeing you!"

You parted ways then, for the last time, he headed for London, you for Dublin.

As the plane taxied out of O'Hare and rose skywards, you watched the buildings shrink, then dissolve. Smiling to yourself, you thought of that strange clairvoyant back in London. How wrong he had been. And the wondrous realization floated up to awareness like a birthday balloon, *I've finally made peace with my past. I could die now!*

Less than two weeks later, you did.

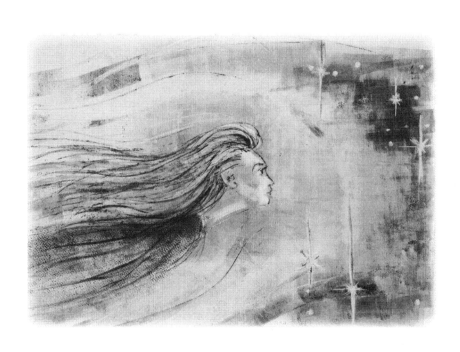

Book 3

THE POETRY OF LOVE

And did you get what
you wanted from this life, even so?
I did.
And what did you want?
To call myself beloved, to feel myself
beloved on the earth.

– Raymond Carver

We believe we have all the time in the world, that the ogre of death won't be daggering his claws into us just yet. Sometimes we can even feel immortal. It's an arrogance and we all fall for it. Even me, strolling back to my room on campus that sunny July evening. I was enjoying my cushy job teaching at Dublin University for the summer. My students' papers tucked under one arm, a scone and jam for supper in the other, I was walking along the footpath and just like that, an earth-shattering thud, and I was dead.

That wild beast, the Celtic Tiger had been growling all over Dublin, proud of its resurrection, and here on campus, bulldozers and cranes were screeching, tearing down buildings to put up new ones, now that the country was flush for a while.

I had heard the grinding engine of a truck behind me, not paying it much heed. It was moving fast, too fast, but I was safe on the path. Next thing I knew, a searing strike to the skull, slicing my breath, and in an instant, I was a rag doll, propelled through the air, limbs skittering. And the world went black.

Suddenly, I seemed to be hovering above everyone else, a bird watching a scene that once I would have considered horrifying. There was a woman splayed on the concrete, blood spewing out of her head and people screaming and calling for ambulances on their cell phones. I couldn't understand what all the fuss was about.

All I could feel was this creamy love – though love is too small a word to contain it – like nothing I'd ever known, saturating everything in its embrace. I tried to tell the grieving people that everything was fine, that this whole apparent debacle was happening in utter perfection, that there was nothing to worry about when every single atom of existence was suffused in this indescribably luscious love. But no one seemed to hear.

As for the broken woman, her papers strewn around her, her scone now a hundred tattered crumbs, she meant nothing to me, just an illusory shadow, an actor in a gripping play whose role had abruptly terminated.

I – whatever I was then – was in some kind of heaven, floating above the drama, free, light as air, brilliant with light, with love, with a profound peace that seemed to say, *All is well. All is well.*

It wasn't until later, when someone in the ambulance slammed a musket of oxygen onto my face, that I jolted back into that shattered woman's body, and the sinking feeling arose, *Oh God. It's me.*

I learned much later that the truck had been carrying huge lumber logs which hadn't been secured properly and the driver was going at such a clip that when he went over a speed bump, the entire load slid sideways, flying off the trailer and crashing into my cranium.

At the hospital, I wove in and out of consciousness, vaguely hearing the ambulance driver telling the doctor in E.R., "It's a miracle she's still breathing. Those were some heavy logs."

The boon of morphine briefly engendered a fit of humor in me. There was a moment when the director of the university stood before me, weeping, distraught, next to my mother, calm and contained as ever. I asked them to tell me a joke but couldn't keep my eyes open for long. I heard Ma lamenting how my looks – whatever they were – would be gone forever. No man would ever look at me again. Even then, I could almost smile at her priorities.

Weeks of vomiting followed, agonizing pain, hours of crying. When I was finally able to limp to the toilet, people would stare at my face, glass embedded and glued to my cheeks with stale blood. The lower lid of my left eye had migrated south. I looked like the reflection you see in those distortion mirrors. Nothing fit together neatly any more. Passersby would sneak a glance and then look away quickly. Maybe it was the morphine, but I found it intriguing. I'd note how long someone would stare before turning away, embarrassed.

Eventually, I was moved back home, into Liam's old room and the cold boulder of reality set in. Posters of Arnold Schwarzenneger glutted the walls and the dresser was piled high with tools and dusty cassette tapes. There was nothing welcoming about it. I lay in bed, staring at the ceiling, wailing for my old life back, the one I'd so carefully built, now shattered into smithereens. I'd hear Mum's voice from her bedroom, shouting, "Stop crying! I can't bear it."

I tried to memorize poems but nothing would stick in my head. I'd grit my teeth and hiss over and over, *Death Be Not Proud*, as if I could fend off the dark knight with the wizardry of language. I was weaving between worlds. I'd try to say *lilac*. I could see the purple blooms clearly, almost smell their heady scent, but when I spoke, *lettuce* would stammer out of my mouth.

I'd lie in bed, a blur of images floating, and then out of this mist, she appeared. Grandma in England. She'd been dead for almost twenty years. But now her face was radiant, soft, so kind. I'd not been close to her when she was alive – she lived in a different country and visited rarely – but here she was now, beaming love at me. I was ecstatic to see her. *Grandma*, I'm not sure if I was really speaking. It was more a language of the heart. *What do you need?*

Nothing, she smiled, light sparking off her. *Eileen, I need nothing.*

She seemed to come to me in my darkest hours, offering love, like a warm blanket I could snuggle in. And then she was gone.

Da was livid as I'd ever known him. He kept talking about the driver of the log truck and saying it didn't have to happen, that he should be put away for being so careless. The driver was the least of my worries. But I'd no strength to say anything, just let Da rant on and on. At least he'd sit by the bed with me. One night, he put a teddy bear next to my pillow and propped an open book in the bear's arms. It was called, *When Things Fall Apart*.

"Go ahead, Eily, have a good cry. No need to hold it all in."

I was surprised and grateful to have permission, though I couldn't have helped it. I'd become a river, weeping, gushing out of me all the sorrows of a broken heart.

One day, I asked Da to read me a poem. He found an old book of mine and began his deliberate recitation. *Prayer*, it was called. And no doubt, it's why he chose it. But a line in it stopped me cold.

"Read that line again, Da, please."

It was almost impossible to be here.

God, here was someone who'd been through the ringer, just like me. *Almost impossible.*

It was the word *almost* that got me. I think it saved my life. Someone else had fallen into the abyss and had not only survived, but they'd triumphed over it enough to make art out of it.

I whispered that line to myself over and over. *Almost* impossible, but not entirely.

For months, flowers and cards and little gifts poured in from America. People I barely knew, former students, Overeaters Anonymous friends, yoga pals, people from the literary world, sent letters of condolence, get well wishes, trinkets to buoy my spirits. There were so many flowers that Ma got angry. "I'm not taking another bouquet in. There's not a single vase left." The sitting room had become a florist's shop. But I was numb with shock. All those stark, pale buds hinted of death. I might as well have been witnessing my own funeral.

Even the editor in New York who left a message to say he'd be publishing the novel I'd worked so hard on had no impact. If someone had told me I'd won the Lottery, I'd not have cared less.

Eventually, I could make it downstairs to the kitchen, though food tasted like sawdust. My body was in constant pain, but it was my insides that really hurt. Though no one could take it away for me, I was desperate for a loving touch, for a word of encouragement. When I reached out to Ma, she flinched and pulled away.

When Da came waltzing in the back door, all rosy cheeked from the cold, he plopped a kiss on my head and said, "D'ye see what a fine day we have, love, just for you?"

"See?" Mum's voice shrill, staccato. "You have your father. The two of you are like peas in a pod. You don't need me."

All the pent up hurt inside me barreled out. "I *do* need you. You're my *mother!*" I pushed Da away and felt badly afterwards.

"You have your friends in America."

"They're not my mother, for God's sake!" We had a blow up row, during which Da sidled out of the kitchen, and the heat.

And then Liam came home for a visit. A family reunion had been planned, long before the accident. We hadn't all been together for years. But the planned outings were a disappointment to everyone. Da wouldn't go if it interfered with his church duties. And every bone in my body hurt when we drove over the tiniest crack in the road.

I spent hours in the back garden. There was a single wild rose in bloom on the bush by Kelly's wall and I inhaled it like it held the answer to the universe. That something so beautiful and delicate had blossomed out of winter's bitter chill moved me deeply. I was out there, drinking its sweet scent when Mum appeared. "Liam got tickets. We're all going to the symphony tonight."

"Oh, good." A trickle of anticipation at the prospect of a change from the constant round of tears, medicine, and more tears.

"Not you."

"What d'you mean, not me? I'd like to go." I was tired of being trapped in the house all the time.

"There's no room for you, Eileen."

"Of course there is…"

"No," she was firm. "Breda's coming too. It'll be too tight in the back seat for you." I watched in shock as she went back inside.

All those years of working the Twelve Steps, I'd trained myself to look for my part in any conflict. But as much as I examined my behavior in the past months, I couldn't find anything I'd done wrong. If I'd known it then, I would have quoted Stanley Kunitz as solace. *The heart breaks and breaks and lives by breaking.*

Some wonderful friends and colleagues in America had opened a bank account in my name and suddenly, I found myself in possession of a lot of money. What would I do with it? I spent a small fortune on gifts for Mum, especially after she got sick and Liam had her admitted to The Mater.

I hobbled the four miles to the hospital, my left arm still in a sling, my body in torment, and offered little gifts to her, a necklace, her favorite 4-7-11 perfume. She hardly glanced at them, shoving each one under the bed. That was nothing new, really, but when she oohed and aahed over Liam's measly Twix bars, I winced.

"I'll get some flowers for when you come home." Surely she'd like flowers.

"No!" her voice was sharp, piercing. "The doctor says it was you put me in the hospital. I overtaxed myself taking care of you. He said I'm not going home until you've gone back to America."

I tried to shove back tears but they wouldn't cooperate so I slunk out of that room and wept the whole walk home.

Perhaps I lived in a fantasy world then, not quite dead, not wholly human. I'd trawl the shops on Henry Street, try on clothes, exotic dresses, cashmere tops, hoping it would make me feel more mortal, more part of the world. But the more I shopped, the less heartened I felt.

The travel section of newspapers became a fixation. I'd read of tropical islands, far from Ireland, and imagine myself basking in the sun, skimming through the water, warm air cosseting my skin. The allure of being bodiless again, floating in pure love, was intoxicating.

It was clear that I wasn't welcome at home and I was in no shape to travel back to America. So I found a Buddhist retreat center, Dzochen Beara, at the southeastern edge of the country. It sat on a cliff overlooking the ocean. They offered daily meditation sessions. But when I saw a photo of giant waves crashing against the cliff wall, I felt nervous. Post Traumatic Stress Syndrome had a hold on me. I jumped at the slightest sound. But it was clear I had to get away.

A local woman, Ruth, had been there and I called her, asking advice, getting the lay of the land. I told her I had some fear about going. "What is it you're afraid of?" She asked.

"The sea. It looks ruthless. What if I'm blown off the cliff?"

She did her best to ease my trepidation, joking. "Well, you can always ring me and then you won't be ruthless any more!"

So I mustered all my courage and took a train to Cork. It was a long, arduous journey. Irish travel is not known for comfort. Then a local bus struggling with a swarm of shoppers and endless bags made stops every few minutes all the way to Castletownbeare, on the precipice of the country. I waited in the town square, wind whipping at my hair, until a taxi screeched to a halt and delivered me to the retreat center. The sky was black as pitch when I arrived.

An affable Englishman showed me to my room. It was clean, spartan. I was so weary, I lay on the bed and listened to the pounding waves until sleep overtook me.

Next morning, I opened the window and gasped at the expansive view. I felt like a bird perched high above the world. The ocean gushed and lapped against the cliff wall, emerald moss tumbling down its back. Surely I'd be safe here.

I chewed on a slice of burned toast and walked up the hill to the meditation hall. A serious monk guided us through a meditation. "Pour two mugs of tea," he suggested, "one for yourself and one for fear. Then pull up a chair and wait."

I liked the notion and carried it with me as I went back to my room. I filled the sturdy earthenware mugs with boiling water and two spoons of tea, the leaves swirling around the lake of liquid as I added milk.

I tried to decipher patterns, read a fortune, but all I saw was two intersecting leaves that looked like a cross.

After scribbling a letter to a friend, telling her I planned to find a monastery somewhere, remote like this, and live the rest of my days in seclusion, I pulled the kitchen chair close to the window and stared at the mesmeric sea.

As day gave into dusk, a glut of bruised clouds elbowed across the horizon. Deep-throated rumbles of thunder fought against the whistling wind. The same monk who'd led our meditation came to my door, a calligraphy of silver streaking the sky behind him. "This is supposed to be a big one. Wrap up warm and make sure your doors and windows are sealed tight."

Oh God, I thought, just what I'd dreaded. I tried talking to myself, offering words of calm but as the wind kicked up and the rains lashed branches against the window, I was in a state of panic. Tea leaves floated aimlessly in the mug of fear.

By the time it got dark, the electric bulb flashed once and the lights died. A commotion just beyond that pane of glass and thin walls was deafening. Trees cracking, smashing against the ground; waves thrashing against the cliff face. I looked for a flashlight. Maybe someone out there would sit with me, distract me from this terror. But if I were to venture outside, I'd surely be blown away.

So I pulled the hood of my jacket up, put on the warmest socks I had and lit a candle. I crawled under the bed covers and read aloud the Tibetan Book Of The Dead. If I was to die again – so soon – I might as well embrace it and recite the prayers they recommended for safe passage. If being clobbered over the skull by a surprise load of wood had been difficult, sitting here in the almost dark with gnawing terror, anticipating the end was even worse.

St. John Of The Cross wrote of the long dark night of the soul.

There had been many rough patches in my years on this earth but that night and the months of pain preceding it were my version of it. I knew about fear and how trying to avoid it only invited it closer. Here I was with the chance to finally meet it.

Somewhere during those dark and dreadful hours, an exhaustion overtook me. I couldn't fight it any more. There was nothing to do but give up, surrender this life to God, wherever he was, to let him have me. I kept reciting the prayers until the candle went out. And closed my eyes, not knowing if I would ever wake again.

But instead of darkness behind my lids, I found an exquisitely beautiful woman. She was dressed in Tibetan robes and her eyes held the sparkle of stars. She beamed at me and that profound peace and love I'd felt when I'd briefly died flooded my being, the room, every atom of space. I longed to melt into her, this stranger who had appeared in my hour of need. But she just hovered before me, offering her magic.

So this must be it, I thought. Death luring me home again. It couldn't be escaped. But the serenity in this woman's countenance soothed all fear. I inhaled her beauty, thanking the gods for this radiant companion who'd ease my passage. I sent love to everyone I could remember, Mum, Da, Liam, my students. And gratitude. *Goodbye cruel world.*

Next thing I knew, the dawn light brightened the room. It was almost morning. The storm had passed. I stumbled to the window. You'd never have guessed the wildness of that water just hours before. It was so calm, you could almost swim in it.

In complete awe, I walked back and forth across the room, to make sure I was really still alive. And then I opened the door. A mess of downed trees, branches, litter, lined the road. It was a slag heap.

Group Meditation had been cancelled because of the weather so I went to the bookshop. And there on the shelf was a book with a picture on the cover of the very woman who'd appeared to me in the night. I was astounded. I grabbed the book and raced to the cashier. "Who is this?"

"She was the spiritual wife and secret consort of one of our great masters. Khandro Tsering Chodron."

"That's a mouthful," I laughed, delighted to have this vision of loveliness literally come to life.

"Do you know the Tibetan Book of The Dead?"

I nodded. "I was reading it all night!"

"In it, it's said that she's the foremost female master in Tibetan Buddhism."

"Wow!" I blurted out my vision or dream but the man seemed unmoved. "Oh, I can imagine she would be capable of that."

I bought the book and left, climbing over the storm's detritus, as I happily planted a great big juicy kiss on the lips of my new and beautiful friend.

Back in my room, the two mugs still sat on facing chairs, like shy lovers. I'd forgotten all about them. When I picked the fear mug up, the cold liquid was clear. All of the tea leaves had floated like sediment to the bottom, not to be seen again.

Months of pain piled up behind me like lead weights. As soon as I could manage, I booked a flight back to Oregon. Some friends had stored my belongings in their garage, my apartment forfeited because I was away so long. I picked up a mug that I'd loved but it felt foreign, like it belonged to someone else from long ago. I couldn't drink out of it. Nor could I use any of the furniture that I'd gleaned over the years. Nothing was mine any more. I had traveled to another world and there was no going back.

So I gave everything away, a free-for-all for anyone who wanted remnants of my old life. I was too afraid to drive so generous friends or taxis ferried me to look at new places to live.

I wanted simple, needed it. Everything had been stripped from me and though it felt raw and vulnerable, it also felt good and in some strange way, right. I considered shaving my head, relieving myself of that burden that made me woman and thus, part of the human race. I longed to peel everything down to its raw essence, just as I had been shorn. Poetry offered a haven for my heart, the way it distilled experience to its roots. No excess, no artifice, just the bare bones of life articulated concisely. I sank into it gratefully. In the world, with its rampant materialism, I was only a bit player, a partial ghost.

A friend helped me find a new apartment. It was in the basement of an elderly lady's home and it perched right over the Willamette river. I was thrilled to have a room again of my own, even if it was bare. Slowly, slowly, I acquired a bed, a table. The spareness suited me. I spent most of my days standing on the porch watching the water flow slowly, steadily past.

My landlady, Betty, eyed me up and down when we met. She was upset that the realty company had accepted me as a tenant without her permission. But over time, we got to know each other. She appreciated my cards that accompanied each month's rent. And I was in love with her garden. As spring woke up, cherry and apple blossoms decked the driveway. Creamy pink magnolias lit up the path to her door. And oh, lilies too and iris and by May, the heady perfume of lilacs and roses wafted through the air as I passed.

If my senses were in Paradise, my body was in hell. The pain in my hips and the length of my left side caused me to limp along, often trailing behind a pensioner twice my age. I tried Watsu, floating in warm water at the local rehabilitation pool, swishing in the balmy liquid in the arms of a strong man. He said the trauma in my body was palpable. I wondered how long I could tolerate such pain.

People were kind. They offered to drive me places, to shop for me. But I was in my own world, a phantom still. Even though it aggravated the pain, I preferred to walk for miles in the rain, in the wind, just letting the elements do as they wished. I was a wispy tendril with two mismatched stalks for legs. Who knew where I belonged?

I wasn't interested in relationships or food or the pleasures of this world. I'd made peace with all the men of my past. What was left for me to do? It was time to find a monastery somewhere and dedicate the rest of my days to God.

Of course, God had his own plan, as I was to discover.

I received the gift of a session with a chiropractor in the northwest. I appreciated the kindness but I'd had too many sessions already and they were grueling. They seemed to patch me back into place for a few hours and then the jigsaw fell apart again. I was weary of trying.

But my friend insisted. She said this man was a healer too and she was certain he could help me. So she drove me across town and I reluctantly went into Peter's office. He was a man about my age, maybe a little older, with radiant blue eyes and a kindness in his manner that engendered a kind of peacefulness inside me.

I shared my story with him, including my plan to become a nun and give up the world. He listened carefully as he made a few gentle adjustments and then sat me down in a chair opposite his.

"Ella," he spoke quietly, "your plan to give up the world is a noble one but I must be honest with you."

I gave him a quizzical look.

"It feels to me like running away. Why don't you face the world, embrace it, and see what happens? You may have made peace with your past but you've not made peace with yourself. The monastery will always be there." Underneath the shock of his words, I felt an undercurrent of truth though I said nothing.

And so despite my misgivings, I found myself traveling across town every Wednesday, asking myself what on earth I was doing.

It felt as if a hand from some other world was gently pushing me towards him. Mostly we sat and talked. I couldn't bear what felt like the brutality of a chiropractic treatment.

And then, Kiara, my old pal from Dublin, called. It had been years since we've spoken, decades. She'd heard about the accident. She said she'd gone to see a fortune teller who told her she had a close friend who was in grave danger.

"I knew it was you, Eily. I could feel it in every bone of my body," Kiara hissed into the phone.

"You *have* to see a doctor *now*. I don't care if I have to take a loan out to pay for it. Promise me – or I'm not hanging up – that you'll do it."

I was desperate enough to agree. And I took a taxi to see Doctor Goering, who was an osteopath. I'd read good things about him and I knew osteopathy was gentler than chiropractic work.

The visit turned out to be fortuitous. He referred me for x-rays and it was determined that my left leg was significantly shorter than my right. Somehow my hips had re-arranged themselves after the wood clipped me on the head and I'd landed in a heap on the concrete. My hips hung on a sharp diagonal. All this time, I'd been lugging this body around with a shortened appendage. No wonder I'd been in such agony; my whole body was torturing itself trying to compensate.

Months of weekly visits ensued. Gentle adjustments and the unspeakable gift of a shoe lift, which evened out my hips, at least to some degree. The pain slowly dissipated.

When I told Betty, she nodded. "I didn't want to say anything but when I met you, the first thing I noticed were your hips were tilted at a shocking angle." She sighed. "I couldn't believe you were actually able to stand up."

I rang Kiara to thank her and tell her the good news. And then she shared hers. "I'm a grandma now," she laughed.

"You can't be! Sure, aren't your boys still in school?"

"Eily," she said slowly, "I never told you – but I'm telling you now! Remember when I left school and went to live with my auntie?"

"Sure I do."

"Well, I'd gotten pregnant. You know how it was in those days, all hush hush. I had a son, Eily, gave him up for adoption."

I inhaled sharply.

"Don't worry. It's a long time since. Anyway, I tracked him down! Michael Dempsey's his name."

"Wowee!" was all I could muster.

"Yeah, he has all the same habits as me, even smokes the same brand, can you believe it?"

On she went, telling me they'd gotten together several times, had a drink and a catch up. He'd gotten married young. "And just last month, he had his first child. A baby girl. Imelda! So now I'm a granny!"

I whooped in amazement and delight. "I always wondered what became of you."

"Well, now you know! And you owe me an ice burger next time you're home. You on?"

"I am! An ice burger and a great big hug it is."

Weeks passed before I learned that Peter offered meditation sessions. He explained that Satsang just meant a group who sits together in silence and observes what arises inside. And afterwards, he would give a short monologue and let people ask questions.

The Friday night Satsang took place near my home so I walked there and lay on the floor in front of him. I still found it agonizing to sit for any length of time. I remember a painting on the wall of soothing, green rolling hills. It was in India, I think. And I loved to imagine each hill was a finger of some loving being reaching down to stroke me.

"There's nothing you have to do," were the first words Peter spoke. I sighed in relief because I wasn't capable of doing anything.

Much of what was shared didn't make sense to me. In truth, nothing really added up any more. But still I came and absorbed the peaceful aura that suffused the room.

As fall inched forward, Peter announced that he would be offering a retreat in Mexico. He felt it would be a very powerful time for me if I chose to go.

The notion of getting on a plane again and riding over rugged roads to get there seemed daunting. Not to mention that one arm was out of commission so I couldn't really swim. It would be torture to be by the sea and just look at it.

Somehow, whatever Peter said, even if I didn't want to hear it, always felt right and true, as if his words were coming from a source other than this world.

And so I found myself in November 2001 in a small village in the north of Mexico. My body was wracked with pain after the long journey. But the play of sunlight on the water opened my heart. Such beauty after such a dark time. I was enthralled. A woman I barely knew said she wanted to go swimming and I threw caution to the wind and peeled off my clothes and we waded into the water together. Oh, the balm of the warm liquid harboring my broken flesh. It was ecstasy.

And when we got to the house where the retreat was to be held, my heart brimmed with joy at the profusion of flowers everywhere and the open courtyard with towering plants. I stood in the courtyard, drinking it all in, while everyone chose rooms for themselves. By the time I could move, I found only a dark room in the basement with shutters that wouldn't open. But I didn't care. I was in Paradise. Amazing how relative life is: after the grim cold of Liam's bedroom and Ireland, this was heaven.

But Peter would have none of it. He insisted that the man

who'd taken the master bedroom trade rooms with me. He said it would be a needed humbling for this man's ego, as he always got what he wanted. I was stunned to be ushered into a palatial room with its own verandah, looking out on the verdant mountains in the distance.

Several days later, I tracked in sand from the beach and was feeling embarrassed about the mess I'd made in such a lovely house. I found a broom and was busily sweeping away the remains of my mess one-handed when Peter arrived. He took one look at me and took the broom from my hand. "Let me do it. You don't need to do anything."

I burst into tears at such generosity of spirit. Having so recently come from a place where my very being was discounted, I was astounded to be welcomed in such a loving way.

That night as we began Satsang, I was lying on the floor, watching the candle light flicker on the photograph of Ramana Maharshi. I knew little of this Indian sage, other than he was the father of the non dual teachings. The idea being that we humans are not separate, lonely islands onto ourselves – that is, dualistic – but that we all arise out of the one source and so are intimately stranded together, like jewels on the necklace of existence.

The more I studied the soft round of his face, the more familiar it felt, as if I'd known him, intimately, forever. I kept staring, lost in the liquid of his kind eyes, and somewhere in the recesses of my being, an image arose. That Face at the foot of my bed when I was a girl. The Face that had offered warmth, goodness when I was at my lowest ebb. The one that had disappeared for decades, along with most memories of my past. Here it was again, the same vision of love, pure, unconditional, beaming at me as if it was only yesterday since I'd last seen him. The hairs on my arms prickled. My heart thudded wildly. It was like falling into Home, that cosy, safe cocoon we all long to return to.

Out of the depths, I heard a voice. The man who'd traded rooms with me was speaking to Peter. I was in a virtual trance and only heard the last words he said. "Praise God."

Something erupted in my chest, a blinding flash of light, of knowing. It was as if the revelation of ages had been placed in my palm. I felt Ramana airlift, quite literally, into my heart and I thought, if it was a thought, that there was nothing more vital to do in this life than to praise God, who'd conjured such incomparable beauty and grace, who'd sent a messenger of love when I'd most needed.

Tears, fountains of tears, gushed out of my eyes, my face a waterfall of liquid. Howls issued out of me: I just couldn't contain them.

"That," said Peter, "is the sound of the heart breaking open."

Next day, I found myself out in the desert, on my hands and knees, overwhelmed with the magnificence of every single thing I laid eyes on. I stuck pieces of jewelry into crevices as gifts in gratitude for this miracle flowing through me. The curve of a donkey's ear enchanted me. Each cactus revealed its secret. The sand between my toes was an elixir of sensation. I was smitten with the entire universe.

Though Peter saved me supper – there was a plate of tortillas on my bed – I couldn't eat. It seemed a waste of time when I could be in prostration, praising every atom of God's creation, which was only another name for love. It was what I'd been born for, in hiding all those long years, now in ripe flourish. I was already full, nourished from within. Nothing was needed. Absolutely nothing. Gratitude was too small a word to describe the joy I was experiencing. I felt as if I'd never lived, really lived, until then. Everything was alive, vibrant, radiant with beauty, from the roughest stone to the expanse of azure sky. And there was nothing separating me from what I witnessed. In fact, it was all me, issuing out of my own bursting heart.

Every agony I'd endured until then seemed paltry, insignificant, and absolutely worth the suffering because it had culminated in this ecstatic illumination. I was floodlit from within, just like everything else. It was akin to experiencing the world inside out, not me floating through the world but the world flowing through this vessel of love that used to be me. I couldn't stop crying, not even to rest or sleep. I was melting into oneness – the inseparable perfection of every single thing.

And Ramana, oh Ramana, who had until now, been a face and a story, a virtual stranger, he throbbed from within, an ache so delicious, an orgasm of the heart, full and rich and all encompassing.

One evening, Peter called me into his room and sat me down. "Ella," he spoke quietly. "It's important for you to know that often, when people have a great opening of the heart like yours, they mistake the source."

"What do you mean?"

"Well, students fall into this deep well of love at Satsang and believe it's the teacher they're in love with."

"You can't be serious."

"It's happened many times since I've been teaching." Peter sighed. "And I just want you to know – as I tell everyone in your situation – that it's not personal. What you are feeling is the presence of the divine."

"I already knew that!" I was stunned. I'd never been drawn to Peter other than as a wise being who guided my spiritual evolution. I wasn't even interested in men and even if I had been, he was not my type. "I don't have any, as you call them, personal feelings for you."

He exhaled slowly, almost with relief. "Well, that's unusual but I'm glad. In case it should happen, please just know that I'm only the puppet, helping you to rediscover your true nature."

I left his room, feeling strange. After that, I was more aware of his presence as we all sat together in silence for meals. And once, taking a walk in the desert, I saw him a few steps ahead of me. An urge to go after him and walk side by side in this ocean of love arose in me. But I quickly quashed it, feeling uncomfortable now, unsure if he'd mistake my gesture for something more than it was.

Next morning, I was up before dawn, strolling along the sand, in awe at the soft crimson sunrise, tears streaming down my face. Peter appeared out of nowhere. "How are you, Ella?"

I stood speechless a moment. "I'm in love." I smiled, gesturing at the expanse of sky and sea.

He looked at me strangely. "With who?"

"This!" And I flung my arms out to the heavens, my heart brimming with delight. "Everything is so gorgeous."

The subtle tension in his jaw softened and he walked on, leaving me to my love affair with all of creation.

That evening, lying on the floor at Satsang, candles flickering gently on the wall, Peter finished his monologue and one by one, everyone left. I was glued to the ground. I thought if I never moved again from this spot, I would be elated. Who knows how much time went by, perhaps hours. The crickets and frogs were conjuring a symphony through the open window. I watched the candle light swirl on Ramana's picture. It was as if he lived inside me, not in the tiny 6 x 8 inch frame. My heart could hardly contain the immensity of the love barreling through my being. I wept and sighed and wept some more. I was Home, here in the quiet, unspeakable joy dancing off every single atom of space.

And then Peter came back in and sat on the floor, asking me how I was. Couldn't he see? I was shorn of words. All I could do was let the tears river down my face. He stroked the damp strands of my hair away from my cheeks, so tenderly that my body began to shake.

He put his hand on my open palm and our fingers slid into each other's. I wanted to kiss everything, even him. I wanted to put my mouth next to every last syllable of this exquisite life. I pulled at his hand, planting bird kisses all over his wrist, still sobbing like a child. Which I felt like, born into the first flush of life's endless bounty. I was thrilled to have someone to share this overwhelming love with, someone who surely understood what was far beyond words.

"You're radiant," Peter whispered.

The candle light shimmered on his face, the ceiling, the walls, until it all blurred through my tears into a lake of beauty, softened of edges. Gradually the light dimmed until it was almost dark.

"It's past midnight," Peter offered. "We should be thinking about sleep."

It was the last thing on my mind. Everything that was ever needed was right here, right now. He started to unweave his fingers. How could I let sleep separate me from this enormity of emotion?

"Stay. Please." This was the most beautiful moment of my entire life. Whenever I'd felt the love of God, even as a child, I was always alone. Here now, I had someone to partake of the beauty with me. It magnified everything.

Peter gently pulled his hand away and left the room.

It's a truism in spiritual circles that someone's big opening is the honeymoon period, the heart expanding, luring the seeker more deeply towards God. And like with any marriage, after the heady wedding days, the true work begins.

And for me, soon enough, it did.

I came back from Mexico renewed, re-invigorated to the possibilities of life.

After Satsang one Sunday, Peter asked for a moment with me. He said he could feel Ramana's deep love for me, and that as he'd surrendered his life to the Indian sage years before, he was being asked to take care of me.

In the weeks that followed, I felt as if I were a wild rose finally unfurling its petals. I didn't need – or even want – anything to be different. I didn't need Peter's help. He lived and breathed inside me. I took long walks through the woods, only this time not to get away from the suffering. I was heady with love, with promise.

Still, Peter left long, loving messages on my answering machine. One morning, he called to say, "You know, it's wonderful this opening you're having. But it will close again."

"Impossible!" I couldn't believe that such expansiveness would yield to anything less than that.

"It's the nature of life. Contraction always follows expansion."

I refused to accept his words of wisdom. Until the hammer finally hit. And it hit hard.

Peter called one afternoon, suggesting he come for a visit. You'd have thought I'd be pleased but I was scared. What if Peter wanted to spend more time, get closer? Even though he was deeply affectionate with everyone, still the notion engendered unspeakable terror in me. I just wanted to lick flowers and Ramana's picture and bask in the love. I kept a photo of him in my bra, as close to my heart as I could get him. It had all felt safe when Peter was at a distance, loving me from afar. I'd been living in my own sweet dream bubble, content with being alone.

He arrived with a fish stew he'd made. I couldn't eat it because of my allergies. He sat on the couch, closer to me than felt comfortable, always loving, light-hearted. I'd seen him lean lightly into people at Satsang, close enough to share each breath. Intimacy was his trademark; he offered love easily. Even though I'd heard him speak often about how everyone craves love, deep down, but if it's really offered – unconditionally – they're afraid of it. And I was scared: I'd run from intimacy as far back as I could remember. The more we connected, the more my fears heightened. There was only so much closeness I could tolerate, who knew why? Eventually, I asked him to leave, feigning fatigue.

Peter arrived again a few days later. He seemed on edge, that light easiness he usually wore dimmed a bit. Autumn was melting into winter. The air was chill. We bundled up and walked through the woods until we found a bench to sit on.

I was savoring the falling leaves when Peter leaned forward and almost whispered. "I'm hesitant to say this, Ella, but I have a strong feeling that you were abused as a child."

I tilted back in my seat, suddenly quaking like an aspen in the wind. "You can't mean…"

I'd shared some stories of my past with Peter and even in Satsang, how I adored my father and had wished to marry my brother. And how for some reason, unbeknownst to me, my mother had excluded me from her affections.

He nodded. "I just ask you to look inside yourself and see what arises. Don't take my word for it."

We walked home in silence. I lay on the bed, each breath shortening, catching in my throat. It didn't take long before a barrage of images, like a movie in fast forward, cascaded before me. A woman, not my mother, leaning over my pram, shoving sweets into my baby mouth, and the deathly smell of feces oozing out of my bottom. And her rage at the mess. A hasty hand shoving the pram into the cupboard under the stairs. The forsaken girl screaming into darkness. Gnawing hunger grinding in my belly.

And oh my father, whom I'd idolized, sought permission from to marry someone else, worried that I'd let him down by having an abortion, the man I'd virtually given my life to – he appeared like a giant, his swollen man tool stretching my baby gums to capacity, his hands rupturing my insides. I watched the little girl – and felt as if it were happening now – as he threw her onto the hay bales at Aunt Lily's and wrenched her uniform up to her waist and found his opening.

I lay on my bed for months, and relived every grueling second of those years. How could I have forgotten the way he found his way to my bedroom night after night and satisfied his hungers or alleviated his pain with my girl body? And how every morning, he got up early and prayed and insisted we do the same. Never a word spoken about it. Where had those years of youth been shelved? Had he erased them from his memory too?

An old photograph I found seemed to proffer a partial answer. It was of Da and me, beaming into the camera, on my last visit home, both of us adults. I'd loved how happy we appeared and had shown it to Peter. It stunned me when he pointed out, in disgust, the placement of my father's hand. It was directly on my breast, both of us blissfully unaware of anything unusual.

Long nights followed, awake in bed, shivering, poems pouring out by the dozen on paper scraps.

My Father's Nipple

My father never gave me away.
I gave him
everything, flesh, love, skin,
the monotone
of my tongue.

I was his bride after the first one,
she who delivered me to him
like one more piece of mail
she couldn't lug on her frail shoulder.

But I was young and bonny then
and married to the world
I found in his rustic eyes.

I imbibed his vows through the open
vessel of my mouth, nectar stream
he caught my fishes in, each furious
release undammed from some deep

> grief in him, he fed his griefs to me
> like Sunday sweets – oh, holy nights
> he groped the peak of his zipper
>
> and unleaked his love in one full flush
> and then another – oh holy night of starry skies
>
> besieged by cloud and lullaby
> in the hew and hush of transubstantiation;
> his and mine, between us we conjured
> water from his wine, we wed our need
>
> in communion. I was his private bride,
>
> the worm in the apple of his heartbroken
> eye, I was his lover, mother, long lost child.
>
> Like this, wholly groomed in our libations,
> like this, we died. And lived.

And more images searing through the canvas of my mind: me in the back seat of my godfather's car as Da left me with him to do what he would. The same with Father Lamb, his thick hands soft as a woman's but brutal in their handling.

One morning, Peter sat me down on my couch. "You know how everyone's original trauma replays itself over and over?" I nodded.

"And how the same situations and patterns keep recurring – different people, different clothing – but bringing up the same wounds?" He'd discussed this at length in Satsang.

"Well, these early dynamics are playing out for you, only now – because you're ready – with the purpose of healing them completely."

"How do you mean?"

"For you, Ella, your father favored you over your mother, right?"

"I suppose he did, yeah."

"And your mother resented you because of it. Hid her anger but resented you, shut you out?"

It wasn't thrilling to hear this. It made me feel like a child. But in ways I was, reborn and still finding my earth legs.

"I'm just a pawn in this," Peter continued. "The same emotions you felt for your father may arise but only to bring them to the surface so they can be embraced. This is about healing the deepest wounds."

I hoped so. I felt like I'd been split open with a razor, all that love that had cloaked my every breath leaking out the holes.

"Ramana has such deep love for you, Ella, to bring you to this place of readiness. It's your chance to really make peace with your past."

Though I would have to slog and struggle through the hell of history for seven years to fully realize that.

After Peter left, I collapsed onto the bed. Barely five minutes passed before the movie started again. Maybe this was how it felt when you finally died – the story of your life in all its minute detail – all those moments long forgotten, unfurling in slow motion before your eyes. Father Lamb, our parish priest decades ago, there he was, in full color, though it was mostly black and white. The sacristy, cold, bare but for the crucifix on the wall. The young girl I was alive again in her starched yellow dress. Him yanking at the skirt, shoving it upwards, rupturing her girl parts with his fingers. Her heart racing – was it excitement or terror? – a scream, hand over mouth, and then – the stench of urine.

One day, Peter suggested we go for a hike in the Columbia Gorge. He'd been an avid hiker in his student days and knew the perfect place. And I needed some respite.

It was a gorgeous, crisp sunny morning when we took off in his red Honda. The entire world was alive, even as a thick nausea glutted my chest. Still, I laughed at Peter's jokes and sang along to the songs he played on the stereo.

We stopped at Crown Point, the pinnacle of a hill, just like its name, with a panoramic view of the winding river and valley below. We asked a visitor to take a photo of us, arm in arm, beaming from head to toe.

Peter led me up a steep hill to a waterfall. I stuck my head as close to its spindrift as I could, the cool water washing away all dross, invigorating every cell of my being. I was ecstatic. We kept walking, uphill, downhill, until we came to a beautiful meadow overlooking the gorge. We sat in the grass, feasting on wedges of cheese, apple, chunks of bread. It tasted like manna from heaven. And there, with the sun smiling on us, Peter proposed a marriage to God, with him as the stand-in. I was charmed at the notion. He presented me with a ring hewn from grass strands. It was more beautiful than diamonds. It would be a marriage to God, he said, to the truth, and ultimately to myself.

In a hilltop meadow, sun streaming down on us, we made a commitment to doing the work together, to rooting out old wounds, and to true, divine union. I wept, those tears born in Mexico erupting again. We invited everyone – the flowers, birds, trees, my family, all of my yoga and writing friends, and of course, Ramana presiding over all of it. The entire world was included in our vows.

As we raced back down the hill, light dappling the soft green of leaves, I was brimming with delight, skipping and leaping through the air ahead of him in delight. "Wow!" I turned back, laughing. "It's almost as good being in nature with you as it is with myself!"

Though this was a huge revelation for me, who'd always favored solitude, Peter was astounded. Only much later would I realize how profoundly I had islanded myself from the world and called that happiness. Contentment. Peace.

Peter would be the one to show me how to open to the human race, how to learn closeness, intimacy, though it would require embracing every remnant fear. I had built a safe haven for myself in the cave of my own company. How would I learn to fully share that sacred place with someone else?

On the cusp of twilight, we approached the final ascent. Though we were both exhausted, Peter hooshed me forward on the hips from behind. It was the perfect metaphor for what was to come: the euphoria of being held, directed forward, loved – and also the complete trust that his hands would not leave my waist and let me fall back into the darkness.

And oh, that darkness draped its heavy cloak around me, a long, coal black night that lasted years. Perhaps the devotion to Kundalini Yoga had enlivened my senses, I'm not sure, or maybe it was the opening of that Pandora's Box of the past but my body was suddenly riddled with sexual energy. An energy I had thought long dead, now resurrected and burning like wildfire. A deep ache, craving release, a bloated dam poised to burst.

I learned to lie on my bed and let the movie of my youth play itself and with each image, the sexual energy would build and as best I could, I let the inferno have me. In our world, orgasm is seen as the pinnacle of pleasure – and in perfect union, it certainly can be – but for me, then, it was a hot, wild, animal clawing at my deepest innards and I was helpless but to let it have its prey.

I would take long walks in the woods, savoring the sunlight flickering on leaves, and then, almost beyond conscious control, I'd find myself straddling a tree trunk. Sometimes I'd have to stop and lie down in the grasses, behind bushes, and let the fire surge through.

One afternoon, when I went out for air, stumbling along the railroad tracks close to my house, a man appeared out of the brush. He unbuckled his belt and opened the zipper of his trousers and juggled his penis out of the opening. It was hard as stone. I turned and ran. That energy – childhood revisited – was so alive inside me now that it was being reflected everywhere.

It seems like an old dream to me now but back then, my body would experience orgasms in the dozens in the course of a day. When the documentary about Doctor Kinsey, the sex researcher, came out, I went to see it. He interviewed people who could orgasm at will, who could have up to a hundred in a single day. I sat in the dark theatre, shivering, knowing that I could have been one of those interviewees.

Back then, my days were a mirage of intensity building, images reeling, pain releasing, a relentless cycle. It was not what one would deem pleasant – especially as history unreeled itself in all its shock and violence – but those few seconds of release were grace, pure and simple. They carried off with them a thread of that horrific girlhood. It was as if I was liberating that pent up sexual starvation for everyone who had touched me, as if they'd only satisfied a fraction of their lust during our entanglements and it was now coming out full flush through me.

It took months of sleepless nights and hazy days, lying on my bed, embracing as best I could a life that had been obliterated from conscious memory. Kundalini Yoga had taught me well. *Allow, allow, allow.* What you resist, as someone wise said, persists. I learned, through Peter's guidance, to open to each memory as it arose, to fully feel the sensations coursing through, and as much as I could, without a story. Just sensation, just energy, however intense, just letting it have its moment of fame and eventually, it would ease and dissolve. I found that wholly inhabiting the intensity that had been so ferocious it had been obliterated from conscious memory led to its dissolution.

In some strange way – later, much later – it engendered

compassion in me for everyone involved. It was almost like panic building and crescendoing into a great white heat until it found its opening and release. But even then, it wasn't done. It was never, ever enough. Sensations of sickness, regret, sorrow all poured through the vessel of this body as it writhed on the bed. The self-disgust in its aftermath, the nausea, and all for that tiny pin prick of release. And yet the perpetrators – and I here now on the bed – were helpless but to follow it. It was patently obvious that this unending cycle of abuse was a sick addiction, an illness, a dis-ease. What medicine could cure it but the love of the open heart?

I hewed to the humble prayer of Saint Francis, *Lord, give me an undefended heart.*

And oh, the endless river of tears streaming over that raging inferno – years of them. And still the wild grappling, groping, unleashing. And always the hope that now, finally, *this* time, it would be freed for good.

"You're not going to believe the joy you'll feel when all this is done," Peter would remind me often. I clung to that promise but at times, it felt like a flimsy thread. The layers of history and conditioning run deep and who knew what God's timetable would be? But Peter had laid his heart on the line for me. Though I gave up waiting for the joy, I held that promise close to my chest. If Peter hadn't been so steady, so supportive and true, I'm not sure I could have endured those years. I'd barely been able to the first time they happened.

Peter continued to call and visit and I could feel the hugeness of his passion. Not for me really, but for love itself. His easy affection flowed off him – towards all of life – like spring water. But the more intimately he approached me, the further away I ran.

I remember driving home one evening and thinking if I had to choose between him and Ramana, I'd choose Ramana. I was in love with both of them but Ramana was God. It was he who had graced me, saved me. Peter was a servant of God, but he was human and thus, fallible.

For a long time, it was like a game of cat and mouse. Peter was supremely patient. He said of course I'd choose Ramana, the way I'd earlier chosen a monastery. It was safe. It didn't rock the boat. It didn't elicit fear.

Whereas with Peter, oh yes, much as I adored him, just like Da, I was terrified of him getting too close. It felt like too much, like a fire that would burn me to a cinder.

A retreat in Vancouver B.C. was scheduled and Peter and I were to travel north together. We'd decided to stay over somewhere on the way to break the journey. I found a sweet houseboat on the Washoughal river in Washington.

It started out well. We laughed and joked and Peter with his usual charm and humor leavened the air. We sat out on the terrace of a cafe in the sunshine and drank iced tea. All was well with the world. Love flowering the air.

But that night, as we settled into the houseboat, that old gnawing terror arose. Every time Peter moved his face towards me, smiling, I flinched and drew back. What was this abject fear? Hadn't I been affectionate with men before? But as I'd learned on this winding road, it was now smacking up against some core piece of childhood wounding. I still needed to protect myself.

Suddenly an image of Ma reared its head. She standing in front of the mirror, swiping lipstick across her mouth. Twirling around in her skirt, inviting compliments. And all of us, me, Liam, Da oohing and ahhing at her elegance. And the unspoken cardinal rule: Look but don't touch. My god, I'd imbibed the same philosophy. Enjoying the admiration, the sideways love offered by men, but rarely letting them near me. The apple, as they say, doesn't fall far from the tree.

All night I lay in the dark, shivering and neither of us could sleep. Peter left the couch and sat on the edge of my bed, gently stroking my hair. After a long internal struggle, my body finally yielded to Peter's arms. He wrapped them round me like a warm, motherly blanket. His tenderness, his unconditional love seeped deeply into my pores. Finally, a man offering himself wholly, the breadth of his heart and love, asking for absolutely nothing. Weak and raw as I felt, I quaked and howled in his embrace like a lost child finally allowed to come home.

Next morning, our host delivered a thermos of coffee and warm muffins. I had a dip in the icy river and emerged, my heart singing. These were the things – comforting food and cold water – that felt safe to open to. A man with the fire of God in the same space with me was a completely different thing.

It didn't escape our notice – in fact, we laughed about it – that the boat was called Karma House.

Once we got to Vancouver and the retreat began, things felt easier. I'd lie on the rug next to Peter as we meditated and he spoke and answered questions. For a few days, a mild peace settled but then one night, out of nowhere, Liam appeared in my awareness. The brother I'd been so enamored of, wanted to marry, there he was, taunting me, bullying, cursing. I was on the floor, savoring the silence one minute, and the next – out of nowhere – screams piercing the room, coughing, sputtering, choking. I didn't realize it was me making such a racket until Peter kneeled down before me, trying to help, and I yelled ferociously, "Get off me! Leave me alone!" Arms and legs flailing as I watched the rope descend and my girl neck thrust inside it.

Poor Peter – I don't remember if I hurt him but I was beyond help, overtaken by the nightmare movie in my head, one I couldn't for the life of me shut off.

EXPIATION

When the body swung
like a question from
the rope, neck become
hourglass snug
in its tether gnawing
raw grit off her skin,

legs billowed, head blown
wide open with stars,
electrified, more vivid
by far than the night
sky which folded over

her like a caul
she could see through,
shades of midnight,
of no escape, of breath
seeping through pores
sapping cells

until she forsook
her own flesh, let
her arms dangle
like puppets, limbs
dripping tears
of sweat, she no longer

needed that moon burst
of god song clouding
her ears and chest,

she was already free,
already melted, o so
quiet, so exquisite
into the deep.

Driving home from Vancouver, Peter and I had dinner at a bright cafe on the waterfront. By then, most of the intensity had lifted. At least for the moment. I was grateful for these breaks, which were rays of sunshine filtering through coal dark clouds. When I caught sight of a group of elderly people sitting on the deck outside, the wind whipping at their wispy hair, I fell in love. I'd always had a soft spot for older people. They had lived long enough to have shed most of their baggage and they were savoring what precious time remained. Without thinking, I raced out to greet them and to tell them how beautiful they looked, like glittering stars in the firmament of life. They laughed and introduced themselves one by one, while Peter watched from inside, smiling.

On the final leg of the long commute, Peter slid a CD into the stereo. "There's such passion in you, you're not even aware of it," he said. "This song seems to be the story of your life." I listened as Van Morrison – whom I'd always admired – sang his hymn of fire.

> *You wiped the teardrops from your eyes in sorrow*
> *As we watched the petals fall down to the ground*
> *And as I sat beside you I felt a*
> *Great sadness that day in the garden*
> *And then one day you came back home*
> *You were a creature all in rapture*
> *You had the key to your soul*
> *And you did open that day you came back to the garden.*

The mix of melody and emotion ripped my heart wide open. We listened and hummed and I cried the rest of the way home.

Peter used to tease me, saying whether I was happy or sad, I would cry. The tears were a welcome release. I remembered Katherine, my old roommate, asking me, in the old days, why I never cried. All that suppressed emotion was finally free to unleash itself.

That joy Peter had promised seemed an eternity away. So many layers. Every time there was a sense of completion, another monster would rear its head. I was weary, worn down, but not defeated. In time, it became apparent that it was the protective ego shell that was dissembling, crack by crack. And oh, the ego fought to survive, to maintain its – false – sense of control. It was an out-and-out war, ego vying against Truth, and I was a mere chess piece in the process. The ego is built to survive; it is an endless denial machine, poised for battle at the slightest movement towards its destruction.

Although I was still eating three meals a day, hewing to the Overeaters Anonymous protocol, my body seemed to be shriveling. You could see bones protruding everywhere. People thought I was anorexic. The doctors claimed that head injuries burned more calories in healing than any other part of the body. Peter said it was because deep down, I felt I didn't deserve to live.

It was akin to living a life in stereo: the normal, everyday life of the present coupled with and mostly overtaken by the life I'd suppressed. I knew enough to be grateful, having this chance to relive my youth, this time to experience it fully – even as poems of anger still poured out night after night. I had to do something with these feelings that were rocking me to the core.

Now I understood why my mother had pushed me away. I'd been a substitute wife – or lover – of her husband's. Whether she knew about it or not, she obviously sensed our connection, which some would have construed as unusual closeness. All the pieces of what had puzzled me for years began to fit snugly – if uncomfortably – into place. Everything began to make sense.

That wild child I'd once been erupted into life again. Without thinking, I began to eat food with my fingers instead of a fork. I could only manage soft, creamy foods. For a while, I bought baby food, apple sauce, and licked the jar clean with my tongue. Flowers in their innocence called out to me and I would lean over their delicate petals and lick them slowly. They were unencumbered nourishment to me.

One morning I rang Mum in Dublin and asked her – begged her – to sing me a lullaby. There was a longing deep within for the nurturing that had been absent in my early years. But Mum, whose own mother had been unable to even lift her up, had never learned the art herself. She couldn't even sing Happy Birthday. When I broached the request for a lullaby, she was stunned, thought I'd really gone off the deep end this time. She suggested I see a psychiatrist. But I had never felt more alive. Raw, certainly. Vulnerable, definitely. As the tears that had been pent up for decades and clogged my existence unleashed, I felt an enormous weight lift. Even with all the pain and grief, I knew I was finally being liberated.

SONGS MY MOTHER TAUGHT ME

"   "

and "   ...!"

Her beak was always busy,
bird eyes green as moon
she built no nest in.

Her hair was spindrift,
no stray twigs
could stick to it.

Her arms were seaweed,
well, that's my dream,
their scent did send me
reeling

but in truth, her whole
body was a trunk
of steely pine,
and nothing

could snap her
silence. She kept
her lullabies to
herself, tucked

safely in
the envelope
of lost girlhood.

The only place
that could forage
a tune was her feet,
the brunt of each heel
as she dashed from
grocer to tea table.

If I had a song
to teach my mother,
it would go like this,

"Sad bird, won't you come
down from your perch,

it's dawn now, and I have
something to show you."

Peter was impeccable in steering me towards the larger truth. And one day, there it was: after years of virtual solitude and meditation, finally, a flicker of light. After a long, profound sitting, a feeling of huge love rose in my heart for my father – compassion too. I saw how wounded he'd been, how powerless, how I'd been his one, warped sense of comfort.

One night, I had a vivid dream, or perhaps it was a vision, of Uncle Jack attacking my father from behind. I barely knew of the word 'sodomy' at that point. But that's what it was. And it explained so much of his behavior. Violence, abuse begets violence, abuse. It's passed down from one generation to the next.

Perhaps this opening to it inside me was a way to end the cycle within my tribe. No wonder I'd never married, not found a man who lived up to my father. A classic case of the Stockholm Syndrome, where the victim falls in love with his or her kidnapper. Mum always said I was just too fussy about men.

It was around this time that Peter proposed a retreat to Ramana's sacred mountain, Arunachala in South India. As a teenager, after a profound awakening, Ramana had heard the name Arunachala and fireworks went off in his head. He decided there and then, by whatever means possible, to go to that holy mountain that conjured lotus blossoms in his heart. At age sixteen, he dropped out of school, left a note for his mother and brother without saying where he was going. And he traveled by train and foot for days to the mountain that would become his own guru. He never left Arunachala for the rest of his life.

I couldn't imagine traveling so far, feeling as fragile as I did. But I still had some money and when Peter suggested something, he was usually spot on. So a small group of us took off one January morning for the holy land, a place where it is said that if you circumambulate the mountain on a full moon, all of your sins will be expiated.

The bus ride from Chennai airport was rugged, to say the least. Taxis, cars, trucks all seemed to feel they owned the road and they made no apologies for it. Horns honked, sirens blared, every vehicle traveling at lightning speed, completely unconcerned about screeching past within an inch of an oncoming truck. It was the middle of the night as we rode and the air was warm and humid.

Stalls selling chai and fruit lined the roads. It was electrifying to be in such a wild, vibrant place.

And oh, that first sighting of the mountain, it took my breath away. Wreathed in shades of jade and bronze, it seemed to drop out of the sky like a gift. Despite the traffic noise, we traveled the rest of the way in silence.

I was smitten by the entire spectacle – and that's what it was, a wildly colorful, ear-piercingly loud display. It felt like a theater, really, God's play, that rolled out its carpet in the morning for its daily performance and furled itself back into the ethers at night.

I was unprepared for the multitude of people begging. I'd been warned ahead of time by Peter not to give my money away. I had a habit of doing that – in fact, a large part of the generous settlement I'd gotten after the accident had been used to help those who needed it. And here, there were so many emaciated people, some of them missing a limb, all with their palms out, following your every move. It was heartbreaking and hard to resist dropping a rupee or two in their hands. But I learned my lesson when I gave a large note to an elderly man who slept in the doorway of our hotel. He waited for me every time I came and left, now accompanied by what I assumed to be his family and friends. Someone told me that many of those asking for money came here intentionally for the winter months as it was tourist season.

The food there was staggeringly good – spicy, rich, pungent. I savored every bite of curry, every mouthful of mango lassi, every last drop of sauce. For two days, that is. After that, I was flattened by an intense stomach bug. I spent most of my days hunkered over the hole in the floor that posed as a toilet. I could barely get from bed to bathroom without a flood of diarrhea assailing me. I felt weak, listless, sad.

I couldn't bear not being on the mountain, and despite Peter's urgings for me to stay close to the bathroom, I trailed after the group as they trekked around the holy hill, having to stop every few minutes to squat by a bush. I was in good company. Countless

Indians used the mountain that way themselves, as a matter of course. It was humbling to see such desecration in such a sacred place – by myself as well – but Peter assured us that the divine lives in all things.

Weeks passed and I was quickly losing weight I couldn't afford to lose. Peter came to my room one evening after Satsang and said, "You look like Jesus. I can see your ribs jutting out through your top. You need to do something or you won't be around for long."

I'd always been stoic about my body, almost forcing myself to see how much pain I could endure. And I was stubborn. But Peter's words, as always, rang true. I was down to raw bone and the diarrhea was not letting up.

So I finally went to the local pharmacy, explained my symptoms, and was duly given a remedy that eventually cleared things up.

By some divine miracle, we were invited to have one meal at Ramana's ashram. It was a strikingly beautiful place, decked in palm trees and flowers. A huge hall with life size photos of Ramana lined the walls. I fell to my knees the first time I entered, completely swept away by the air of peace and love. My senses drank it in like the scent of jasmine.

When I looked up, it was straight into Ramana's eyes, soft, tender, kind eyes that bespoke a love I'd not felt since I had died. As I sat there, almost in a trance, a bolt struck my chest. That Face that had visited me as a child – when I was most vulnerable – rose up again. My beloved Ramana! He'd been with me all those long, miserable years and even through the times I'd forgotten them, forgotten him, forgotten God and yes, myself. It felt in that spectacular moment that I was looking into a perfect mirror. Who could say where one reflection ended and the other began? It was one, harmonious, beautiful whole.

Out of the air, I heard softly but distinctly, *You are my first and chosen one.*

I sat for hours, lost in love, in joy, in gratitude. It was only at Peter's prodding that I made it to the lunch room in time for the most delectable, nourishing meal I had ever eaten. Ramana had insisted on feeding the poor every day. And a half century later, here I was – o lucky one! – sitting cross-legged in the same room as he once had, scooping luscious heaps of dahl and sambar and yogurt and sweet rice off a banana leaf with my fingers.

Though the body was still weak, a yearning in the heart tugged at me. I had to climb to the crest of Arunachala, just once, to follow in the wake of Ramana's feet. He said that there wasn't an inch of his beloved mountain that he hadn't set foot on. I'd heard it was not an easy ascent but I also knew I wouldn't rest until I'd attempted it.

I hired a local man, Subramanian, to guide me and we set off in the middle of the night, the moon lighting our way. How to explain the feeling of being lured upwards, as if a firm hand was nudging me forward, step by precarious step. Sweat drenched my clothes but my heart was singing. We stopped periodically to sip on water and rest on a rock. And just as the sun was peeking out over the mountain's crown, we reached the top.

A flood of ecstasy washed through me as I stood on the precipice, wind whipping at my hair, the whole world fanning out below. In a flash, who knows what possessed me, I had torn off my clothes and stood arms raised to the heavens, naked before God. For that brief moment, everything dissolved, the heartache of this life, the torments of the flesh, that long, winding, arduous road to here.

Subramanian, perhaps embarrassed by my rash display, discreetly turned away while I melted into infinity. Never had I felt the heart-rending magnificence of pure existence. It was a moment I would tuck into the deepest reaches of my heart and cherish forever.

Only much later did I recall the clairvoyant in London's prediction. He had been right after all. I had fallen madly in love with a mountain.

Before I left that magical land, another beautiful gift presented itself. In deep meditation one day, I could feel Da as if he were sitting beside me. Still the images of him rifling through my clothes, unearthing his treasure, floated through with all the attendant unease. But now I saw with the clarity of crystal that perpetrator and victim are two ends of the same spectrum – each feels powerless: one tries to overcome it and the other becomes helpless, but they are both victims. It is one thing to understand this intellectually but quite another to actually experience firsthand the truth of this. When it finally dawned – like a long awaited sunrise – I could feel only sympathy and sadness for the brute trap of my father's life, for the insatiable hunger of my godfather, for the priest who must have wrestled with profound guilt, and for those sorry friends of Liam's who had to hide behind a shield of false power. And for all those predators out there – despised as sick and brutal by the larger populace, and probably as lonely as a human being can be.

And still: when I returned to Oregon, it became clear that it was necessary to share the truth of my experience with Ma and Da. Having always tried to protect them from pain, the notion brought up intense trepidation in me. I sat with the deep discomfort for a long time and Peter helped me through the thick of it. Weeks, maybe months unfurled, until finally I picked up the phone and dialed their number.

WHEN I TOLD THEM

He said, No, never.

She said, I know him
better than he knows
himself. He never would.

Girl On Fire

He said, Food is important
and, Are you warm enough?

She said, It must have been
somebody else, someone
the help brought in.

He said, It's terrible
what happened
in Auschwitz, but they're
apologizing now.
Pope John Paul
comes from nearby.

And where is he
with his condolences?

She said, Who can
blame the young Germans?
They weren't even there
when it happened.

And your brother,
Yes, I can imagine
his friends might
get up to mischief.
But we're saying
nothing. You speak
if you must.

He said, I'm going
to Mass. I'll
offer it up for you.

Why not light
a candle too
for all of us?

And the heart cried,
and the throat choked
back inside its noose.

And two doves flew
into the seedling tree
on the bank, and
paused a moment

before one flapped
his wings, bored,
restless

and the whole branch
snapped.

The conversation was never mentioned again. It was as if it hadn't happened at all, just like our entire history together – or apart.

Several weeks afterwards, I was shopping for Christmas presents. In the haze of the ever-present past, I'd lost track of time. I was barely functioning in the world. But I wanted to get gifts for Peter and my landlady. It was a crisp, sunny day and I saw a bakery on Burnside. Two women were sitting in the window over mugs of steaming coffee. It looked so inviting, I thought I'd run in and buy a cuppa, warm myself and hopefully get a boost of energy.

I had an urgent need to pee so I raced into the bathroom. The toilet door swung wide open and then came hurtling back at an alarming rate and crashed into my temple. I reeled backwards, stunned, until I could uncoil some toilet tissue and press it soaked with cold water on my forehead.

Feeling nauseated and sore, I decided to skip the coffee and go home. By the time I got to my front door, my eye had swollen and a bruise of glorious colors – green, turquoise, vivid red – was forming. I looked like I'd been beaten. Hard.

Although it throbbed intensely, at times I forgot about it. A few days later, I went to New Seasons, a notoriously friendly health food store. The cashiers usually had a warm word or a comment to share. As I laid my purchases on the counter, the woman turned to smile at me and then caught sight of the rainbow hues around my eye. She quickly looked down and away, taking great care not to make eye contact. At first, I was surprised at her swift change in manner.

But then the truth dawned: she thought I was a battered wife or something and was embarrassed. I wanted to tell her I'd simply walked into a door but then thought better of it. Why would she believe me when most of the world saw a woman maimed and thought the very same thing?

The acclaimed Irish novelist Roddy Doyle had written a novel about an abused woman in Dublin. He called it *The Woman Who Walked Into Doors* because that was the excuse she always proffered when she had to appear in public with her black and blue face. I'd taught the book, for God's sake, in my novel writing course. Back then – or so I believed – I had no personal relationship to abuse.

But now I fully understood what it felt like to be judged, dismissed, even pitied. I could feel the hollowed-out space in my gut where self-esteem used to live. As one of society's dregs, I was finally feeling the despair and heartache of those long years of violence. It amazed me how supremely kind the universe is, allowing us, when we are ready, to revisit the events in our lives we once needed to eradicate, in order to survive. When we died a little – or a lot – to ourselves. And here now, I had the chance to hold that injured, broken girl in my heart and love and accept her completely, unconditionally.

Slowly, slowly I learned to see beyond the intensity of that regurgitated life. I began to feel again the perfection that guides every atom of existence, just as I'd felt when I'd died. And the love permeating all of it, excluding no one. Who could I shake a stick at, really? Everyone who'd visited horror on me had been deeply wounded themselves. They were looking for love, for relief in the only way they knew how.

And then, years down the precipitous, winding road: a miracle. Out of thin air, a vision or perhaps it was a dream. It felt more vivid than anything I'd ever deemed to be real. One night, ensconced in my cabin on the Oregon coast where we were on silent retreat, a man – a being, more accurately, definitely male – appeared. How he found his way into the room was a mystery. But I wasn't afraid. He had a silhouette that felt old, familiar but the votive candlelight dimmed everything. His beautiful wraithlike body hovered over mine as he slowly, tenderly drizzled his fingers along the contours of my skin. He could have been a ghost, so translucent he was. The hairs on my arms bristled with fear, or excitement, who could say?

I lay still, drinking in the milky warmth of his hands, the way he knew just where to touch me. My heart – and body – felt wide open as he dropped bird kisses on my eyelids, cheeks, neck. My hair was liquid in his hands. In the flush of twined fingers, of warm skin on skin, it took a moment before I realized he had found his way inside. How to describe the intimacy, the divine beauty of such coupling, tongue swirling round tongue, teeth sharp on gum, heart pressed to heart, the slow, steady rocking, building, building – it was like drinking pure mountain water after years in the desert, a heat flooding the room, a power far beyond anything known, and a wild flush of divine nectar swimming, electrifying every cell, every orifice, places I'd not known existed until now. And a scream – was it me? – riding out on the air, piercing the stars.

When I woke next morning, the room was cold. No lover snuggling next to me. But the peony buds on the table had blossomed during the night – a chalice bursting with ruby charms.

I was freed. I knew it as clearly as I knew my name. That old beast of past violation had finally been slain. I lay in bed, touching my skin in curiosity, as if it had just eased itself anew out of the dark womb.

For weeks, the visions wove in and out of consciousness, as if I were in a delirium out of which I'd wake eventually. But it was an exquisite madness, an almost beatific gift – the astounding marriage of human and divine – bestowed so mysteriously and received so gratefully. Dream versus reality – who could say which was which? Certainly not me. Certainly not then. For those exquisite moments, the dualities, the opposing forces, the extremities of polarity – dissolved into a sinuous, unspeakably bountiful, delicious whole. Nothing felt separate or apart from my own heart or body.

STUDIES IN LIGHT

The world is full of mountains.
Arunachala, speak to me.

The world is full of beauty.
Shiva, shine on me.

The world is full of lovers.
Ramana, make love of me.

Every evening
as stars peel back
the skin of sky,
he comes to her door
and slips inside
and his fingers
find her heart

even in her fever
in her quaking legs,
he makes her shiver
through the heat of skin
and bone pressed
in the nameless dark
together.

> Each night,
> he delivers seeds
> for her to plant
> in her unprotected center
>
> to which she adds
> water in the morning
> and a leaf, a petal,
> a psalm of green
> swim in its reflection.
>
> Each twilight,
> she lies in her room,
> heels pinned to the mountain.
>
> Now, when she parts her legs,
> she sees God.

I rarely spoke of all that happened when I had that near death experience. It felt too sacred, too intimate, perhaps. The perfect love, yes, the peace and joy, that was easy to express. But one piece of it had always puzzled me. After I discarded my body and floated off into infinity, I remember encountering a series of dark caves. I knew there were beings inside and in the way that 'dead' people communicate, wordlessly, I asked each of the beings if they would take over for me – I still had my students' papers – as I would be gone for a very long time. And I remember how not a single being volunteered to come out, much less assume my life, despite my impassioned pleading.

In that moment of profound disappointment, I realized there was no one who could do the work intended for me. I had no choice but to re-enter that battered body.

And one day, many years down the road, I understood. The beings hidden in those murky caves were aspects of my own consciousness that I'd buried in padlocked chambers of my heart. In the process of making peace with myself, which Peter had advocated, one by one, each dark cloud emerged and revealed itself. The miracle – and it still feels wholly miraculous – was that once I fully opened to and welcomed each memory and the excruciating emotions that accompanied it – they dissolved. Literally melted, ice in sunshine, floating away forever.

HIS

When I fell in love with God
I was so besotted, I wanted
to eat my way back through
the earth to Him, the way
my father tried to eat me,
meat of the world, groin,
limb, thigh, foot, locking
sucking chewing biting
grinding down to ash

whatever gives under
all that force, that
revived passion
without boundaries

that hews to no one's
rules, that lives and
dies and loves every
last flower, stinking

weed of the fields.

It took seven long years but eventually I emerged from my inner cave, light as air, as if I'd shed a great weight I'd not even known I'd been carrying.

Yes, I cried for several years straight but they were tender tears, the heart breaking open wider and wider so it could contain more and more. I could now feel the extremities of what it is to be human. I sobbed for those I'd never met who had suffered. A newspaper story of a murder or a child's terminal illness would have me weeping. And on the other hand, my heart exulted in the scent of a wild rose, the shy smile of an elderly woman. This was what it meant to be fully alive, fully present to the vast dichotomies of this existence. In contrast, I realized how profoundly anesthetized I'd once been. When I looked back on it, that existence felt like cardboard, brute survival, a quarter life.

I understood more deeply what the Passion of the Christ meant. How suffering is a doorway, if we open to it, one that yields unimagined treasures. I knew I could never go back to that limited, predictable range of emotion.

I began to feel the enormity of others' grief as if it were happening to me. I was no longer a separate, suffering individual without hope. I was part of and profoundly connected to each jewel on this necklace of life. Amazing as it was, I began to see those years of meeting the pain head-on in a way I couldn't as a child as an enormous blessing.

Gratitude may seem like a strange word for so many years of torture but I was – and am – supremely grateful for every second of it. If my life had been a bed of roses, I may never have found my way back to God, to myself, to the true, undivided heart of love.

But along the way, there were startling moments, as I watched repressed patterns reveal themselves once again. When Da had his first stroke, he was in a coma for several days. As soon as he came out of it, the first words he uttered – to Mum – were, "Where's Eily?"

Mum said she told him I was in America. But I didn't miss the disdain in her voice.

I went back to Dublin several times after that. The first visit, Mum greeted me at the back door with a *You look well,* though how she could have known that is a mystery, for her sea green eyes darted in every direction except mine. They rarely landed on her daughter, as if the sight might be too much to bear.

Daddy was still in the Mater hospital but he was in good spirits and we sat and chatted as I cried next to his bed. It was as if my revelation of our yoked history – years earlier – had never happened. As I was leaving, he asked me to hoosh him up and hand him his walker so he could escort me down the corridor.

As we waited for the lift, I found myself fondling his pajama buttons, opening them all the way down to reveal his white chest hairs. He smiled, a sheepish look on his face. It was something I'd done with lovers in the past and though it shocked me, I was helpless to stop it. Finally, after a long, loving goodbye, I buttoned him back up and fled down the back staircase, my heart racing.

Back in America, I took to calling him often. He'd share his usual jokes and we'd have a laugh. And he'd ask me questions about my life, my writing, things he'd never been interested in before, hadn't had time for. Now he was roped to a hospital bed and had all the time in the world.

He'd always ask about the birds where I lived. He'd befriended a robin in the back garden before he got sick and he loved to lean over and pet him, imagining himself perhaps a bit like St. Francis.

Invariably, he'd launch into his favorite, Ode To A Skylark. *Hail to Thee, Blithe Spirit.* And I'd pick up the next line, *Bird, thou never wert.* On and on we'd go, stumbling forward through the stanzas until he'd lose a line and I'd sit waiting for him to re-conjure it. As the years went by, he could barely recall the first line. But when he'd get a word or a phrase, he'd be triumphant, as if he'd unlocked the key to the universe. It made my heart sing to hear the jubilation in his voice.

Oh, we were like two children then sharing the bounty, the poetry of our love.

AFTER THE STROKE

He came back for a while,
a fragile butterfly determined
to mend, but the fireworks
in his head kept sparking
and there seemed to be no end
to the thunder in his brain
half silence ten thirds pain
and o his heaving breathing
on the line, I could feel
the chest straining to break
free, to shed its brutal
captivity and fly right
though the wires
chrysalis abandoned
wings in wild expansion
directly into me

The second time I returned was for the court case, to negotiate a settlement for damages following the accident. Daddy was in hospital again. I'd called him several times from Oregon and written to tell him when I'd be arriving.

ADVENT

It was like those calendars
you have at Christmas
tearing off the windows
counting down the days
to the only one that matters.

This is what he said
when I arrived: I was marking
time until you came.

His neighbor said, I've
never seen a man so excited, like
a child expecting Santa.

What his room mate
on the ward said:
He's talked of nothing
else since I got here.

What she said: He's weak
so be prepared.
What I said: Nothing.

My mouth was full
of tears.

Even after all that had passed between us, I still loved him more than any man. The hard edges of raw survival had softened in his face. His normally conservative, suspicious ways floated into the background. When he said his eyes were bothering him from the diabetes, I suggested bilberries as I'd read they were good for the eyes. "Ah sure, why not, love?" He smiled. "Whatever you say."

Ana Ramana

THANK YOU MOON

Last time you were in your prime,
I turned off all the lights in the oratory
and told my father to close his eyes
and drew back the gauze curtains
so we could sit hand in hand beside
each other like secret lovers
and watch your beauty shine
through the glass that named us
Hospital, that called us Jail,
so we could invite you right in
to the room that would tomorrow
enclose him and set me free,
all the way past the label
his wife affixed to him helplessly:
In valid, right on past
the long desperate past
that had so long trailed
us, on through the lonely
shroud of torment
and brute joy,
yoked in that unending
moment

that would dribble
out of our hearts then
and onto the sidewalk
for the rest
of our natural lives.

We sat together like long lost lovers, hand in hand. I massaged cream into his bad leg and he cracked his usual array of jokes. The only awkward times were when Mum arrived and found us sitting perhaps too close together. She said nothing, as was her way, and kept herself busy, unpacking the medicines she'd bought for him. I felt a stab of pain in my chest, though, and wanted to hug her. But she was occupied, doing what she needed to survive.

Once back in Oregon, I received a large padded envelope from Mum. Inside was a delicate silver Rosary with a beautiful sculpted image of Our Lady on it. A curt note said that Da had sent her on an errand, money in hand, to buy this rare piece. She'd had to take two buses across town to pick it up. And he hadn't told her who it was for until she brought it to him. "And what did he buy for me?" she wrote. "Nothing."

I placed the Rosary on the little altar by my bed, though I didn't say those prayers any more. They conjured too many memories that weren't exactly pleasant. Silence seemed more fitting now than bleating stock phrases, though I knew many people hewed to and relied on them.

An elderly man in our parish once presented Da with a Rosary that would take your breath away. He'd carved it himself out of hardwood and each bead was the size of a man's fist. It was as tall as an adult almost, and must have weighed a ton. Daddy seemed amused but a little chuffed by it.

He was never one for gifts, couldn't even remember his family's birthdays. But when I'd last seen him in hospital, he'd handed me a piece of brown ribbon, streaked with gold. "Mrs. Dalton sent me flowers, Eily, but the nurses took them away. We can't have them here. But look, I saved you this ribbon – I thought you'd like it."

And I did. I cosseted the little strip of acrylic between my fingers as if it were the crown jewels. It was the first present he'd ever given me that wasn't religious, that felt thoughtful and kind.

Even though I was flooded with love and understanding for the darker underpinnings of my past, I remained – in heart and body – glued to my father for many years. I wrote him cards with huge flowers crayoned on them so he could see some color, even as his vision was fading. And miraculously, he wrote me back.

Ana Ramana

UNFINISHED SYMPHONY NO. 100

His scrawl like ribs
crushed and crawling
over each other, letters
splashed in almost blood across
the page, his love I suck
off each scratch of
pen through space

and into that place
no one else can touch
after all these years
and all his age
and disease of flesh.

After all, there remains
the funeral march
of alphabets, of time,
that ravages
and saves,
this love still
burning like a lightning
blade, this love given
in some strange god
storm fallen on father,
on daughter, that will

not die, his will to write
to say his hand is cold,
to deny the stroke
that shakes the pen
and quakes the head,

nothing happened,
as if to say, nothing
has changed, our love
remains.

> And he's right.
> I can read the signs
> in the beginningless
> endless, scriptless
> tale of the unwritten page.

As his health declined and he'd had three strokes, he was moved to a nursing home in – appropriately – Oldtown, County Meath, miles from Dublin. He was declining mentally too. He could chat away like his normal self at first, but then he'd throw the exact same questions at you, over and over. Liam grew tired of it. Mum too, though I believe she mostly indulged him.

On the phone, I let him go on and on and on, just delighted to feel the rich connection flowing through the lines. It wasn't in the words but in the joyous mood of our communion.

I still lived in the small apartment overlooking the Willamette river. Hummingbirds flocked to the flowering plants I put on the porch. They whispered of joy, of ease, freedom. One morning as I lay on a deck chair milking the sun, one of them landed on my head. He crawled across my crown, a tiny tickling on my scalp. I didn't dare move but I was smiling like a Cheshire cat.

They became my intimates, these birds, so drenched in color, floodlit by the sun. Such tiny vessels embodying such delight. I bought a penny whistle and tried playing to them. We formed a makeshift duet, though my contribution was meager. I penned poems to them, these glimmers of joy in those dark days.

Betty, my landlady, lived upstairs. She was 85 when I moved in. An ardent Catholic herself, she was thrilled to learn of my father's industrial strength Catholicism. They would always ask after each other and send blessings across the water. Da would often inquire after her, even when his memory was failing him.

Ana Ramana

MY FATHER ON THE PHONE FROM OLDTOWN

after telling him I would plant poppies for my 'poppy'

What color will the poppies be
And when will they grow
And what do they look like
And where are you planting them
And isn't Betty great for her age
And what color is your car
And how many students do you have
And where do you find them
And isn't Betty great
And are there boats on the river
And how do they fish
With nets or
And isn't Betty
And do they get mackerel
And do they keep them
And how is your weather
And how is your health
And where are you sitting
And what color are the flowers
And

When will you call again?

I received one final letter from Da. And it shocked me. The envelope read, *Eily Massey. Portland. Oregon. USA.* No street number or address. No zip code. He was barely in his body. I imagined him straining to write even that much: the letters were scratched onto the paper in a dizzying display. Inside, the yellow sheet of lined paper held one word, written in huge, sprawling letters. L O V E .

I kissed each magic mark passionately, tears seeping out of my eyes. Ramana had said that tears flowing out the side of the eyes meant joy and in this case, he was not wrong. I'll never know how that letter reached me but I bowed in my heart to whoever had the wherewithal and knowledge to deliver it to its rightful owner.

Over the long months, Mum kept me up to date on Da's progress – more accurately, his decline. He slept most of the time. She said she'd found a pamphlet in his bedroom that shocked her.

"HOW TO BE CELIBATE"

You'll need to rummage through
the piles of paper in my father's
gutted room. Gutted because
he does not sleep there now
under wads of newspaper,

gutted because the life he lived
under that roof has burned out,
gutted like this heart that heard
his wife say, "He wanted something
so I sifted through, and this is
what I found: He'd sent away
for it, God knows why."

She said the first imperative
was to stay away from women,
don't even enter the same room.

And somehow his wife took up
his cue and sent him packing
so she is free in her vacant nest

and he, the shell of him, keeps
time in that nursing home
in Oldtown, so far away
it takes two buses and a taxi
to reach.

So each of their wishes
has been realized. God is good.
And mysterious.
Amen.

She said she'd gone to visit him just last week and he was half awake. He'd asked, like a child, "Who's that you are?"
"Don't you know me?" Mum had asked.
"You've a lovely voice." He'd replied and drifted back to wherever it was he lived now.
Though Mum took it in her steely way – stiff upper lip – and said, "I'm fine," it tore at my heart hearing that she was hurting and he was folding more deeply into the tomb of himself.

ODE TO MY FATHER'S NIGHTINGALE

Come back! Come back!
Circle his head with your wings
like a halo in shades
of the earth you both
came from.

Please don't
rest your song – not yet.
There's a perch for your weariness
on the branch of his ear:
Please, please sink your beak
deep in its whorl, thick
now and dull as death.

Pour your sweet liquid back
into the holes in his skull,
note rising on note in a swirl
that will unsettle his torpor and let fly
the poem trapped
in his heart.

Speak through him,
I beg you, once more

in a long flow he can hear through the flatness.

Pry open the bud
of his mouth sealed
against winter

and brim with the music
I barely remember,
unceasing, violate,
whole.

I prayed fervently to Ramana to keep Da alive until I could see him one last time. I offered anything, bargained, wept, begged. Underneath, I knew it would turn out exactly as it was meant to but I had to ask – or plead, more accurately.

And mercy of mercies, I did manage one more visit. I'd gotten a teaching job in Crete and though it was gorgeous and my heart sang, swishing in those turquoise waters, I was counting down to D-Day, when I could wing my way across the Irish Sea and rest in my father's arms again.

Only it didn't turn out quite like that. Public transport in Ireland is notoriously unreliable so I was up at first light to walk the three miles into town so I could spend several hours in the freezing cold waiting for the bus that would take me past Swords and onto Ballyboughil. Then I hired a taxi to ferry me to the nursing home in Oldtown.

When I finally arrived, the receptionist was busy chatting and waved me on. The huge, old house smelled of decay, despite the stench of cleaning fluid. The walls of the hallway were scattered with photos of Da below the caption, *Beechtree's Most Famous Resident*. There he was in all the glory of his rugby days. I felt proud.

It took me a while to find him. He was in a small room, in a wheelchair, staring into space. His right hand shook wildly.

"Daddy!" I crept up towards him, a huge grin on my face.

He looked me up and down as if he should know who I was but couldn't quite place me. My heart sank.

"Daddy! It's me, your girl, Eily!"

A few moments plodded by before the light dawned. "Well Eily, if it isn't yourself! How are you at all?"

I sat in front of him and took his calm arm and stroked his fingers to warm them.

"And where is it you're living now, my chailín álainn? America, isn't it?"

I nodded, my throat glutted with all the pent up excitement of seeing him again.

"Daddy, what happened your hand?" It was twitching like mad, never resting. It was a result of his third stroke but I didn't want to ignore it, pretend it wasn't screaming for attention between us.

He looked down at it briefly and said, "It's nothing, girl, only I'm a bit cold."

I sighed, deeply, witnessing or at least acknowledging for the first time how profoundly we can suppress the truth from ourselves. How could I judge him, really, when I'd lied to myself for decades?

THE STROKE

Oil of grapefruit, lotion of roses
I smear across his heels, tender
fingers sprinkling kisses
on each of his endless feet

thick as carcass, nails
tough, yellow, blood dried
between his toes, his age
wafts through the air

in stages, half man, half
mold, all succulence
to my nostrils, this skin
which is my intimate

my own love, foundation
of my father, out of which
his flesh arose and which
softly, gently molds between

my fingers, yielding, supple
almost, as he sinks back
into his wheelchair, smiling,
o sweetest, needed repose

remnant liquid smoothed
on his temples, on the flakes
along his nose, last vestige
caught between our fingers,

o so tightly yoked, his warring
hand freed for a perfect moment
until the stroke regains hold,
his wrist spinning

in crazed circles above
his groin, seat of all terrors,
all regret, ghost of his daughter's
flesh forever spinning

in the web of his upset palm.

When it came time to leave so I could catch the last bus into town, I pushed his chair towards the dining room for supper. Each resident had an assigned seat. I met the man who sat opposite Da, and in that moment, I felt a wave of envy. That he should be the lucky one to share every meal with my beloved father.

But when I leaned down to kiss and hug him goodbye, he resisted, pulling back into himself. He didn't want anyone to see such an open display of emotion. I tried twice, hoping I'd misread his gesture. But no, his head was lowered over his soup and all I heard was a muttered, "Safe home now."

I felt like one of the church women who'd circled him like flies after Sodality, wanting the attention of the holy man they imagined. He'd brush them off quickly, like dust on his lapel, and scraper away. Once when I was with him, Mrs. Quinlan was moving in, eyeing us up and down, "Eamon, who's this lovely cratúr with you?" Daddy grabbed my hand, said, "I'm sorry, Mrs. My daughter's home from America and we're in a hurry." And he dragged me off down the avenue after him, a cluck of curious women staring in our wake.

And here he was now, embarrassed by the attention, even from his daughter who'd traveled across the world to see him. Deep inside I knew that he would have behaved the same with anyone. But my heart was broken. Simply shredded to bits. I stumbled out the sliding doors, sick to my stomach, and threw myself onto the wet grass, howling. Was this to be my last sighting in this life of the man who had possessed my very being?

The bus was late and I missed the connection. I was freezing and my eyes were swollen and raw but I didn't care. I let the tears unleash themselves until I was exhausted. By the time I got back to Ma's house, a scab had formed, the way it does eventually to protect a deep wound.

Ma was beside herself when I walked in the door. "Your father's been ringing every five minutes for the past three hours!"

"What d'you mean?"

"At first, I thought he was ringing for his usual after-lunch chat. But no, all he could say was he wanted to talk to you. I told him you weren't here. But did that stop him? No, he rang every few minutes to check if you were home yet."

"Oh Ma," I didn't know what to say.

"I asked him would I not do? No, he said in that stubborn way of his. I'm just not good enough. It always has to be you." I reached out to stroke her arm but she was already pulling a tea towel off the rack and opening the oven. "You can ring him back. I'm finished dealing with him."

She was shaking though she tried hard to conceal it. I was as surprised as she was. Last I'd seen him, Da had wanted nothing to do with me either.

Sighing, I did ring him back and he picked up immediately. He was all gush and palaver, saying how very much he loved me and how my visit lit up his day and how he needed me to know that. He was falling over himself with compliments and declarations of love. He sounded like someone fighting for his life. Underneath it all, I knew, was a profound apology, one he couldn't quite articulate.

I listened to the words I'd longed to hear for years. But by then, it was too late. I'd given him everything – body and soul – and he'd spurned it. I never saw my father alive again.

I did keep phoning him once I returned to Oregon, but he gradually lost command of his voice, couldn't speak at all. I'd call and beg the nurse to place the receiver by his ear. For hours, I'd whisper into the almost silence, into the ragged hum of his breathing.

On his birthday, I rang three times before the nurse agreed to wake him and hold the phone up for him. I was halfway through singing Happy Birthday when out of the blue, I heard it. *Happy*

Birth-day, dear Eam-on. Happy Birthday to me. I thought I was dreaming but no, there was the deep throaty voice I'd long loved singing along with me. Daddy singing! I burst into tears as I heard him laugh heartily and repeat the song several times.

How could it be? He wasn't able to speak, I'd been assured of that. The nurse took back the phone eventually and said, "Well, isn't he in good form today!"

I barraged her with questions. How was it possible that a mute man could sing? Was he – oh, wild fantasy – actually recovering?

No, she sighed. "It's a strange thing, lovie, but the part of the brain that affects speech doesn't seem to affect singing. Isn't a good thing yer da is Irish now? Sure, we're nothing if we're not a nation of singers."

I hung up the phone and sat staring out the window for hours. This life could be so wild, so intense at times, and yet it offered miracles right out of the blue.

But Da's good spirits failed him after that. Even when I got him on the phone, he would grunt weakly. He didn't try to sing anymore. It was as if that old depression that had long plagued him had taken up residence again. I would wake in the night, feeling the burden of his pain like it was my own, and in a way, it was. An old man, voiceless, trapped, splayed on a mattress in a lonely room, unable to use a muscle except those of his mind. Who knew what torments surged through him those lonely years?

But it felt too, in some strange way, like poetic justice: that I was now free to express the depths of myself to him and he could do nothing but listen. "Daddy," I whispered into the phone, hoping it was soft enough that the nurse couldn't hear. "I have to tell you that I can't be married to you any more. I need to be free."

I could hear him straining on the other end, heaving grunts issuing out of him. I knew he was trying to respond but now he was the child, the powerless one. The ball was in my court and I held it close to my chest. "I love you, Da, always will." I went on. "You're a good man in many ways. How generous you were to me in these last years, walking all those miles into town, leaning on your cane, to get me a cashier's check. And the way you let me cry after the accident. You were brutalized yourself and I'm so sorry for that. But it's time to move on now, do you understand?"

His breath got heavy and fast. I knew he could hear every word. The nurse took back the phone and said, "He seems to be in a lot of discomfort. Maybe we should hang up for now."

But no, I answered. I wanted him to have to hear me right through to the end. Reluctantly, she put the receiver back next to his ear.

"You'll always have a special place in my heart, my poppy," I went on, tears flushing out of my eyes. "You know that. And even though it was a strange relationship we had, I know you couldn't help yourself. You did your best. I wish we could just have been father and daughter, like normal families, Da. But I was your lover almost since I was born…"

If a man in a coma could scream, that is the sound I heard rushing through the wires then. He was desperate to respond. But like me, as a girl, he was powerless but to stay in place and imbibe.

"Please know that I forgive you, Papa. Everything, all of it. There's a rose in my heart that will always be yours. Just know that, okay? But I'm letting go now. It's time for me to…"

An ear piercing sound thundered through my ear and the line went dead.

I tried calling back several times after that but the nurse always said he was sleeping. She said he'd been more restless than usual after our last conversation and that maybe I should wait a while before ringing again.

Maybe he did need time to digest all I'd shared, I don't know. Each day, I left messages for him at the nursing home. "Tell him, please, when he wakes, that Eily called and she loves him with all her heart. Tell him that. With all her heart."

Ana Ramana

EAMON

She'll surprise me, she'll just show up one gray afternoon and light it up in the way she always does, and I'll sit her down, I will, I'll tell her everything that's been buried in my heart, how much I really loved her, even then, especially then, how proud I am of her, my chailín dhilis, and oh, I'll sing for her, all those ballads I should've sung long ago, what matter I can't carry a tune, Danny Boy, maybe, or The Black Velvet Band, she'll like that, 'her hair, it shone like diamonds, you'd think she was queen of the land' and she'll listen, her head resting close to my shoulder, like a bird, and this time I'll pour it all out, saving nothing, all the torment, the night terrors, the agony of lying still, of not being able to hold her, just hold her one more time, and she'll clasp my hand, calm it, soothe it, let it come to rest. 'And her hair, it hung ov-er her shoulders, tied up with a black velvet band.' She'll understand, she will, she has to.

And when it's time, after we've embraced and forgiven all, she'll surely stand here weeping as I float out of the room, the angels lifting me at last out of this terrible body, and I'll wipe her every tear, I will surely, and tell her not to grieve. She wouldn't want me to slip out the back, would she?

And her tears will melt into the river of light, leaving only her eyes, those blue moons that drew me in all those years ago, those I will carry with me, no matter what.

THE LAST TIME

When I call him
for the last time
to tell him
I won't be
coming home again
so he can let go,
the nurse keeps
taking back the phone
to say
how he is struggling
to move, how his
one working hand
is shaking
and his breath
hard and strong
as if he would
leap out of the bed,
she says, in his
longing.

All is forgiven,
I say,
all stains erased.
Lay down
the blame you've heaped
on yourself for all
the roles you've played.

"I'm just a thought
away," I say.
"You live inside
me now."

And after,
sitting on
the river bank,
tears streaming
down, a sound
from the water,
a sea lion
raising his head
and then diving
back down into
the mystery
as a hummingbird
soars across
the sky

the whole universe
saying, good man,
good woman,
you did your work,
*everything is going
to be all right.*

Eventually, Da's leg was so riddled with gangrene that it was decided it would be amputated. I read that gangrene is literally death tissue in the body. He was moved to a hospital in Dardistown. I could feel the life force slowly leaking out of him, his helium almost all expended.

TELL ME AGAIN ABOUT LOSS

My father is on his way
to the place of teeming light.

He is already three-fourths
water. Where then

is room for fear
when he is sparkling

liquid flowing
off that body:

a mere thought
a phantom life

that he mistook
for real, and hurt

him beyond saying?
Now it is becoming

time to retrieve
what he forsook

in place of guilt
and history,

time to melt back
into timelessness

into his exquisite
seamless divinity.

Ana Ramana

EAMON

They're coming for me, the angels.... I can hear them now.... Ah, what a symphony.... A flood of rapture so divine.... Hail to Thee, Blithe Spirit.... Oh, the white of their wings, bird thou never wert, so soft they flow, leaves in a breeze and they're singing my name, my real name, I remember it now, how lovely... how soft, oh, I'm only delighted to go with you, where are we going, will Eily be... ah, sure, I know, it's not her time, is it... ah well, tell her I love her, tell her... let her know, would you, before... whisper... love.... I love you, Eily, mo chailín álainn, my special girl... forgive me, I know you will... purest heart... that girl, don't you see my point, angels, she's one of yourselves, surely, she'll know what to do, her heart's big enough for the past, don't you think so, isn't that right, Eily, sure, isn't that the gospel truth, don't forget me now, will you, don't forget how much you... how much.... I have to go now, don't...

I was on a silent retreat at the coast when the call came. At lunchtime, the cook casually mentioned that my mother had phoned and wanted me to contact her. My breath caught in my chest as I ran downstairs to the phone. I didn't need to hear the words. I already knew. The body that had possessed me all my life no longer existed. And even amidst the flood of tears, I knew deep inside that the heart – his love, our love – lived on.

I skipped the afternoon meditation and went down to the beach. A cold wind had reared up but the sun was out and I peeled off my clothes and ran with all my might into the turbulent waves. The icy fluid felt sharp, comforting. I thrashed through the water, raising my head periodically to scream, who knows what. Something ancient was releasing itself. When I'd worn myself out, I floated on my back, eyes closed, letting the liquid lash against my skin. When I opened my eyes, a sea otter was poised right next to me, his ghostly eyes fixed on mine. He was so close, I could have touched his slinky fur. We gazed in surprise at each other for a long moment before he dipped his head and dove back into the deep. I raced like a mad woman up and down the beach, stark naked, not caring if anyone saw me.

I was grateful for the retreat, for the chance to sit with the tumult of emotion flowing through me. Why hadn't I felt him when he died? We'd been so close. He'd passed at 5 a.m. American time, alone in his hospital bed, the day before his leg was to be removed. I'd been awake then, flailing in the bed, trying not to wake my roommates. But I'd felt nothing. Not a whiff of his slipping out of that garment of flesh I had so cherished.

Later that week, after a particularly profound meditation, I went for a long walk. Sunlight flooded the fields and I lay down on my back in the tall grasses, lit a cigarette. As I watched the smoke spiral skywards, wisps of gossamer, I was struck by an indescribably profound knowing – as if it were written in block capitals in the kernel of my heart: *Nothing Is Mine.* How to describe the feeling of ecstasy that flowed through me, the relinquishing of all protection, of possession, the sundering of decades of effort. I felt as if I'd been freed from a life sentence. The unspeakable burden of hefting all that need, that desire, that sense of *mine, mine, mine.* It was a miraculous moment, sadly short lived.

FIRE, IN PARTS

Whatever I loved, I took inside me.
Every orifice was God's.

My father was the first to come
inside my mouth.
He was a fleshy trout
I suckled on.

But I saved my tongue
for grasses and tall flowers.
I made snakes of them.

The lost boys and angry men,
my bitter brother entered
through the lower cave.

They thought I was a lake
that could ease all heartache;
I made a nest for them.

Birds swam in and out my ears.
My lap was home to starving dogs.

Every orifice was God's.
Whatever I loved, I took inside me
and I loved my Master most.
He taught me to be a glad host
to the dream pain,
to offer my flesh and skin,
to give what I couldn't love
back to Him, until

my heart swelled out of itself
into His heart's ocean

until *my* melted into the mist
of existence.

I didn't go back for the funeral but watched it, bizarrely, on the internet. Our parish in Ballygall had a camera set up for all ceremonies, probably aware that many emigrants would not be able to get home to Ireland in time. For me, there was no point in going back to that place of dark memory. My father lived as brightly in my heart as anywhere. I knew from my own near death that his body now was just a spent skeleton. But that is not to say that I didn't cry when I saw the pallbearers, Liam among them, hefting the wooden box that carried what remained of my father. I blew him a long kiss, my hands quivering, before I turned off the computer.

Mum rang a few days afterwards. She said she was just carrying on, sorting through Daddy's things, getting rid of them. Keeping busy kept her sane. She said she'd found a large envelope in his bedroom. It was filled with every letter and card I'd ever sent him. He'd saved them all.

"Not even a trace of all the postcards I sent him from England," she said sharply. "Not even one."

"Oh Mum," was all I could manage.

Then she proceeded to share, proudly, that she was ordering a marble headstone for his grave that would read, "EAMON MASSEY, LOYAL TO THE END."

As l hung up, I felt such compassion for my poor, long-suffering mother who'd been spurned from day one. And for him too, for the ways he'd had to trample down his fear and passion so he could survive. They both did their best, I believe that, truly, as did I. If we were to do it over again, who knows if it would be any different? I was just grateful that I'd come to a place of understanding, of sympathy for all players, and not just stayed trapped in what I was or wasn't getting from two flawed, misguided human beings.

They happened to usher me into this world and as such, there was an umbilical cord connecting us through the dark blood of our lineage but in life, that cord never united us, only tugged and tore at each one of us, snaring us in its stubborn grip. The only place where true unity and wholeness, free of the bruises of the past, can take hold is in the sanctuary of my own being. And there they reside, intimate parts of my own self, not less or more significant than any other part. They played their role, as did I, and the play, though tragic, ends happily, as each of us is subsumed back into the true heart of love.

ENVOI

Strangely – or perhaps perfectly – after that long, black night of reckoning, I saw less and less of Peter. He seemed to fade, like a vague mirage, into the background. He'd been loaned to me to hold my hand through the murky trail of the past's ravages. I could never have done it without him.

He visited one last time and sat me down. Calmly and lovingly, he told me that now his work was complete. Just like Magdalene, he'd helped wrest the demons clawing to my being. It was time for me to leave the nest, like a budding eagle, and fly free.

Slowly, painstakingly, I faltered my way back out into the world, leaving the cocoon behind. The ferocity of my past took on the aura of a filmy dream from which I had finally awoken. There came a time when I could look back on that wild history as if it were someone else's. It no longer touched me. Eventually I would have a real, lasting relationship with a man, without the baggage of a brutal history dragging us down.

Sometimes I'm overwhelmed with gratitude for all Peter bequeathed. To witness how he surrendered his own will, and let Ramana direct the play, even as we sometimes stumbled round in the mystery of it, inspires me to the core of my being. A famous prayer Ramana once wrote to Arunachala goes, *Let thy will be my pleasure*. Peter embodied, and continues to embody, true surrender, as I slowly learned to.

Peter, from his vantage point of freedom, had shone a mirror at me, a reflection of my liberated, stainless self. His unconditional love, sincerely offered to that broken girl-woman I'd once been, slowly, painstakingly led me towards the limitless, pure beauty inside my own being. Even the feeling of Ramana as other dissolved, melting into my own heart, that universal, singular heart of pure love. After imagining myself smitten with many a man over the years, nothing could have prepared me for the love affair of the ages. The uncontested love of my life turned out to be me.

As we all are, every single being, creature, stone on this planet. Imbued with the divine kiss of perfection. I came to find, in the most unlikely places, the imprimatur of Love, fanned out across this wild, mysterious world, excluding nothing.

EPILOGUE

After my father died, I couldn't feel him. For about a year, I would search for a sign of him, sometimes a dove – his bird, symbol of peace – would appear on my birthday. The dove would settle in the eaves and sing his mournful lament and my heart would break open and imbibe. Then I began to have strange feelings, heaving depression, wanting to die, profound pain in the body. I'd have ferocious headaches, something unknown to me before this. And I'd find myself holding grudges against someone, stubbornly holding on to being *right*. After a while, I realized these symptoms were my father's. That the shell of the ego when it is formed is not only yours, but is the sum of the relations between you and both of your parents, a three-way affair. I had internalized so much of my father's angst, fear, and righteousness, that now that he was no longer in a form that could embody these, they manifested through me.

For three years, I wandered in a haze, flailing, uninspired to do much of anything. I distracted with movies or food until I felt numb. There were moments of such intensity, I felt I couldn't bear it any more. I prayed to God to take me. And somehow I stumbled through if not forward, hoping it was healing something for him.

And then, fours years to the day that he passed, I went to Satsang and an enormous presence arose inside me. Words fall short of describing how it felt. Perhaps the closest I can come is to say that this presence felt like God, the true Self, saturated in love, in light. And into that hugeness, my father had finally dissolved. An overwhelming sense of peace washed over me, like a bath of grace. And just like that, my father was no more. He had vanished into, how can one speak it, infinity.

Tears of gratitude, of all-encompassing love overflowed from my eyes, now seeing the truth of everything. The story of my father – after all the wild wrangling, the collision of love and need, the suffering that yoked us together – had melted back into the source out of which it arose. Not my father *as* Presence but my father vanishing back, subsumed into the all pervasive Presence that he always was.

And as I slowly emerged from meditation, a vision arose: vivid as if it were happening right now. My father at the front gate of our house, white hanky in hand, frantically waving me off as I left for America, his face a sunbeam of smiles. I watched him get smaller and smaller, shrinking until there was only a gossamer hint of tissue waving in the breeze. *Goodbye, dearest girl, travel safe, be happy, goodbye.*

UNTIL SHE SAW

She never knew she used to be
the woman who walked into doors,
and not straight through

her forehead gashed against
the edge as it crashed open,
her eyelid black and blue
and purple as the swelling
spread, a disease of boys
and men no more brutal

with their sticks and penises,
their clubs and fists
than she was to herself.
She learned it from them:

to bludgeon her shell
with whips and falls
that were no accident,
each smash a new badge
of pain to cancel

Ana Ramana

the one before, as if
she could outrun them,
like shadows she legged
it as far away from
as her girl limbs
could. She became

them, she became
an animal, fragile,
clumsy, broken
– and she told
– no one –

until she saw
through eyes
the shade of coal,
twin fires in
the bloodshot whites,
the ash of her past
held in her pupils

until at last she saw
there was no roof,
no walls, no floor.

And she strode forth,
not her father,
not her mother,
not Jesus,

but walking on water.

ACKNOWLEDGMENTS

I owe a huge debt of gratitude to all the wonderful people who championed "Girl On Fire" over the five years it took to complete. This tale of transformation could not have happened without the steady love and unfailing guidance of my spiritual teacher, to whom I will forever be grateful. I also bow to my faithful friend, Prem Caulley, who was my first and trusted reader as I penned my way through these pages. His wise and honest counsel and our lengthy discussions nourished not just the book but my spirit too. Bless you! I am also indebted to the unstinting generosity of my dear friend, Lynn Patterson, whose sustained support has been monumental. Also, a special hug of praise to Jude Burns, whose warm encouragement when energy was flagging reignited my passion for bringing this massive project to completion.

Warmest thanks also to my lovely pal, Pema Deane, who encouraged me to initiate a Kickstarter fundraiser to offer financial assistance while I wrote the book. I was overwhelmed by the massive outpouring of support from beloved friends and people I had never met. I bow to each of your bountiful hearts for your kindness. Particular appreciation goes to my beloved heart-sister, Amrita Brummel Smith, and to Michael Veys and Peter Debilius, for their heartfelt support. I also remain in utter awe of Mark and Maggie Wisdom, who watched the final hours of the fundraiser online, knowing that the requested amount of $10,000 needed to be reached by the set deadline or all would be lost. At the last minute, they and their beautiful friend, Mary Ho, stepped in and brought the campaign to a joyfully successful conclusion. I will never forget such a colossal act of generosity. Also, an extra hug of gratitude to Amaya Villazan, who patiently filmed the fundraising video.

And to all of you beauties who donated to my Kickstarter campaign. No matter what the amount, every single cent was welcome and contributed towards this book you now hold in your hands. Not least among you is my treasured sister, Claire Callan, whose constant love and intimate chats have buoyed me through the years.

And immense appreciation too for the warm, wise and helpful support of the Women's Council, which formed for the express purpose of advising me on matters financial and practical. Bless you, dear Pema Deane, Judy Morgan, Lynn Patterson, Caroline Jones, Jude Burns, Shanti Joy, and especially my cherished friend and confidante, Sura, who conjured the idea of the Council in the first place. My dear friend, Lily Keller, deserves high praise too for her unwavering support and encouragement. Also, a hearty thanks to my beloved pal, Ruthie Hunter, for her boundless kindness.

In 2013, an excerpt of "Girl On Fire" was published in the illustrious New York magazine, "Carrier Pigeon," which fuses fine art and fiction. I was profoundly honored that the brilliant artist and friend, Bruce Waldman, provided breathtaking illustrations to accompany the story. There are no words to express my gratitude to him for allowing me to include them in this book. Bless your kind heart, dear Bruce!

I also owe a huge hug of delight to my beloved friend, Bodhi, who, with her immense graphic design talents, conjured some mock covers for "Girl On Fire" – with Best Seller all over them! – to boost my confidence as I wrote my way through some difficult sections. And I can't forget two wonderful friends who championed the book – and warmed my heart through some challenging times: Kathy Zavada and Kelly Ryan. Blessings too to Lani O'Callaghan, who read and helped edit the finished manuscript.

High praise also to Prem Das and Kira Brooks, who both contributed towards the book's cover. Prem, your keen eye captured the perfect photograph and you and Kira did a marvelous job of graphic design. Kudos to you both. Gratitude too to Aaron Rose, who added a touch of finesse to the book before it went to press. Also, a glad shout out to my lovely friend, Ryan Bouslaugh, who offered welcome advice in the final stages of the book's birth.

Thank you heartily to my lovely students, whose vote of confidence kept me going at times and to those of you who came to hear me test drive "Girl On Fire" at a reading in Portland in 2014. Your feedback was immensely helpful. And huge praise to Kristin Killops for opening her beautiful home for the reading.

As the saying goes, it takes a village. And what a far-ranging, eclectic, generous-hearted community banded together to contribute to the realization of this life's dream. May "Girl On Fire" ignite a flame in your heart, dear friends, as you have, passionately, in mine.

GLOSSARY

Aisling: A dream or vision, often symbolizing Ireland

Bad cess to him: A mild curse on someone

Blinds: Window shades

Cailín Álainn: Lovely girl

Cén chaoí bhfuil tú?: How are you? A standard Irish greeting

Chancing your arm: Testing the waters

Chuffed: Charmed, delighted

Cidona: Cider

Codger: An elderly man

County Louth: The smallest county in Ireland

Cratúr: Irish for "creature"

Dahl: A spicy lentil soup

Dick Whittington: A folktale character who lugs a pack over his shoulder

Dodgems: Bumper cars at a carnival

Dosh: English slang for "money"

Eejit: Dublin slang for "idiot"

Erin Go Bragh: Ireland Forever

Fag: Cigarette

Garda/Gardaí: Policeman/Policemen

The G.P.O.: The General Post Office, main branch in town

Gurriers: Young men who are rowdy, trouble makers

Gye: A concentrated yeast extract paste

I'm only after making apple jelly, etc.: Carryover from gaelic, used often in Irish dialect

It won't always be dark at six: English expression, meaning "Things will get better."

Janey Mac: Irish expression, loosely translates to "Wow!"

Jotter: Copy book

Knackered: Irish expression, meaning "exhausted"

Lansdowne: Famous rugby stadium in Dublin

Leaving Cert: A national exam, the results of which determine your eligibility for university

Like chalk and cheese: Two distinct and opposite qualities in a person/thing

Lorry: An articulated truck

The Mater: A Dublin hospital, meaning "Mother"

Messers: People who joke around, making fun of things

Mitching: Skipping school

Mo Chailín Bán: My White (Special) Girl

Mo Chailín Dhilís: My Sweet Girl

Mo Chroí: My Heart

On the dole: Out of work

Prataí: Potatoes

Primary School: Grade School

Queue: A line

Sasanach: A derogatory term for a Saxon, or English person

Sambar: A lentil vegetable stew

Scarper: Race away from something

Slagging: Jeering

Smithwicks: An Irish brand of beer

Sodality: Catholic prayers devoted to Our Lady

Tannoy: A loudspeaker

T.D.: Teachta Dáil, politician, member of parliament

Tolka: A river in north Dublin

Uisce Beatha: Whiskey

Wellies: Wellington boots

Wired to the moon: Irish expression, meaning "crazy"

The Wreck of the Hesperus: A ship that sank

You'll be better before you're twice married: English expression, meaning "It will be better soon."

You're gas: Irish expression, meaning "You're amusing."

About Ana Ramana

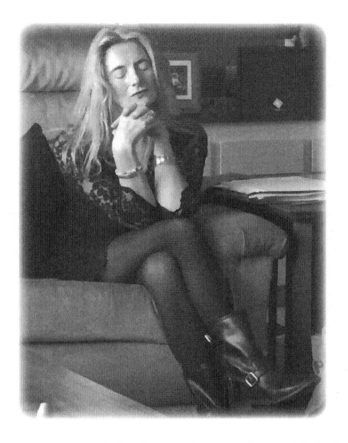

Originally from Ireland, Ana Ramana has published three books of poems and a novel. Her awards include the Academy of American Poets Prize and the Heekin Foundation's Fellowship for Literary Nonfiction. Her work has been published and anthologized worldwide. Publishers Weekly cited her as an Emerging Writer To Watch. Much of her recent writing emerges from prolonged periods of silence and meditation.

She offers intimate Spiritual Writing workshops and retreats by invitation, in the US and abroad. Topics include, but are not limited to, Writing About Family/Ancestors, Grief Processing, and Health/Illness/Bodily Issues. Her students include high school poets, professional writers, the elderly, medical students and faculty, and the terminally ill. She tailors each session to the specific needs of each person.

A variety of clients have also commissioned Ana to write poems for special occasions.

You can find more of Ana's work on her website, anaramana.com, or visit her blog, intimaciesoftheheart.wordpress.com. If you would like to receive a weekly poem in your inbox, you can sign up on Ana's website (anaramana.com). If you wish to invite Ana to give a reading, talk, conjure a special poem, or to offer a spiritual writing workshop, you can contact her directly at anaramana777@gmail.com.

Made in the USA
Lexington, KY
08 July 2019